CAN

A PARAMEDIC'S

YOU

ENCOUNTERS WITH

HEAR

LIFE AND DEATH

ME?

JAKE JONES

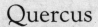

Quercus

First published in Great Britain in 2020 by Quercus.
This paperback edition published in 2020

Quercus Editions Ltd
Carmelite House
50 Victoria Embankment
London EC4Y 0DZ

An Hachette UK company

A CIP catalogue record for this book is available
from the British Library

PB ISBN 978 1 52940 428 9
Ebook ISBN 978 1 52940 425 8

10 9 8 7 6 5 4 3 2 1

Typeset by Jouve (UK), Milton Keynes

Printed and bound in Great Britain by Clays Ltd, Elcograf S.p.A.

MIX
Paper from
responsible sources
FSC® C104740
www.fsc.org

Papers used by Quercus are from well-managed forests and other responsible sources.

In memory of my dad

Contents

CONTENTS

CONTENTS

Prologue

The ambulance is halfway to hospital when Samuel lifts his leg and puts his boot through the window.

It's a humid afternoon and the roads are sticky with hostility, so the driver makes plenty of noise as she weaves through the traffic. But lights and sirens are old news in this part of town and no one gives us a second look. Unless they see that foot.

In the back with Samuel are two medics and a constable. We can't do much about the protruding limb, because we're busy holding the rest of Samuel down on the bed. He's tensing and twisting and grabbing and groaning. He's a fish pulled from the water, a flailing power cable.

It's okay, my friend. You're perfectly safe.

We're on the way to get his heart fixed. When we left he was calm, in a kind of stupor. But his brain's just woken up to the fact it's been cheated of something, and now he's lashing out, rolling over, throwing his face at the floor. And trying to climb out of a moving vehicle one limb at a time.

The window's barely big enough for a foot to fit through: a sliding porthole high above the bed. Reaching a leg up there would be an achievement for a man in the prime of his life.

What makes it more impressive for Samuel is that fifteen minutes ago he was dead.

I

It's there as soon as the door opens. Sour, sweet, stale: it surges down the corridor in search of the outside world. It burns the nostrils and sits like a powder at the back of the throat.

Small breaths, small breaths.

74-YR-OLD FEMALE, COLLAPSED, NOT ALERT

No one is ever alert. This is a truism of telephone triage. Even when they've made the call themselves, no one is ever alert.

We approach the flat. Flies dance in the doorway. The odour thickens, expands, envelops us. It has layers; it has texture. It's a physical thing, a presence, a force-field. A chemical weapon.

In the background sits the acrid infusion of stale cigarette smoke, years of jaundiced fog now seeping back out of the walls, as if the building has emphysema. Then there's the moist undertow of congealed sweat turned rancid like butter, collected over weeks in flaccid pouches of unwashed flesh until the skin turns raw. More potent still is the stench of fermented urine, a restless homebrew, saccharine-rich and vinegar sour, viciously leering. Finally, the sharpest odour of all, the sickly fruit of peptic turmoil, an acidic, rotten tang, almost a taste: diarrhoea.

These are the smells that cannot be unsmelled.

Hello?

Come in, guys. Thanks for coming.

A bald head appears down the passage. Someone else who's up too early.

It's my downstairs neighbour. She's in a bad way.

We step into the flat. The carpets are threadbare and rucked to reveal the concrete underneath. Crumpled council letters, pizza leaflets, food wrappers and tissues litter the floor. The yellow paper on the walls is peeling at the seams, and where the walls meet the ceiling, a dense lattice of cobwebs is laden with thick pillows of dust. The smoke alarm beeps: HEEP! CHANGE MY BATTERY! Every forty seconds: HEEP!

What's the lady's name?

Margaret. Peggy.

A single unshaded bulb illuminates the living room, but the stronger light comes from the giant television. Dominating the centre of the room, like a monarch at court, it pours out a multicolour cascade of the life Peggy could be living if things were different. Its sound has been muzzled to a dull, persistent murmur.

Torn curtains hang below the window line on a rail that can no longer take the weight. The walls are devoid of adornment: no black-and-white wedding day; no grandchildren in school uniform. The carpet in here is not something you see; it's something you feel. As we step into the room, our shoes cling to it like flip-flops on wet sand.

Peggy doesn't have much furniture. On a small Formica table ringed with caffeine haloes sits a glass ashtray, overflowing with butts and tobacco threads and the mouldering debris of miniature oranges and other fruits. Mugs have grown encrusted with dregs, other food waste has been discarded on the floor: yogurt pots cultivating blue cheese and greasy wrappers hosting flies and their maggoty young.

The sofa itself is a broken-down hearse, beginning to fold in on itself, its material balding and sprouting foam, its original colour long forgotten. Surrounding this seat, within arm's reach, sit five or six ice-cream tubs that explain the throbbing stench – because each of them appears to be full of urine.

And in the centre of the sofa, her limbs flopped out exhausted to the sides, but with eyes staring stubbornly in front, sits Peggy.

Morning, Peggy. I think you might need our help.

Every occupation carries its own mythology. This one has the sparkle of excitement, but don't be dazzled. Not all flashing lights mean there's a disco going on.

Perhaps it sounds like an adventure. A little bit daunting, a tiny bit glamorous. The racing through traffic, the unpredictability, the public trauma, the blood. The vague whiff of danger. An exhilarating little escapade.

You see it when people ask what you do for a living. You

say the word *paramedic*, and their eyebrows lift slightly, their heads tilt a fraction to the right.

Oh, wow!

And, just like that, for a moment, a very short moment, you're a tiny bit more interesting.

I could never do what you do . . .

I don't think anyone pictures a permanent adrenaline rush. But there's that tantalising collision between crisis and intervention, especially out in the real world, where local details can add a bit of spice.

You can guess what people ask next. We all have that guilty-morbid fascination with the nasty things that happen to people we'll never have to meet. So of course the next question is:

What's the worst thing you've ever seen?

When someone asks this, they're after a cut-price horror movie. They want to hear about the man who's taken his hand off with a bench saw or the girl with a pen lodged in her eyeball. The more gruesome the better – and preferably involving a large puddle of the red stuff. Tales of mangled limbs tend to be well received; descriptions of organs outside the body elicit luxuriant groans of horror.

What they don't want you to tell them about is the thirty-four-year-old on the second floor with two young children and motor neurone disease, acting out a roleplay with her husband from her mechanical bed to make things normal for the kids. Or the elderly lady who attacks her husband with a stick because she now thinks he's an intruder, while he clings to her wrists and wipes the tears from his cheek with the shoulder of his perfectly ironed shirt. These are not the right kind of 'worst thing'. They're a bit too possible, a bit too wretched, a bit too *real*. Shootings happen *out there*, on a screen, in the news, down in the badlands. Dementia can happen to your mum.

And what they really, *really* don't want to hear about is the woman you had to lift out of her own excrement.

Peggy looks like the wicked witch from a fairy tale that went out of print twenty years ago. Her hair is a ragged rope, with streaks of turmeric yellow. Her skin is like oatmeal gone dry in the sun. The flesh of her face hangs heavy, loose, surrendering in thick creases, out of which peer the defiant beads of her eyes.

I don't want your help.

Why not, Peggy?

I don't want your help.

She murmurs these words like she's reciting a message someone made her commit to memory. Only she's not sure who the message is from, or for. If she was a wicked witch once, then all her evil schemes have long since gone to seed. Though she'd still give a child a fright if they got lost in the woods and wandered into her cabin.

I don't think you've got any choice, Peggy.

We can't leave you here like this.

Won't you let us help you?

Defensively, she reaches out to her friend – the remote control – and turns up the sound on the television. Then drops her arm in her lap. The whites of her talon-like nails are black.

We turn to the neighbour.

What actually happened?

I was leaving for work. I do shifts like you. I heard her call out. The door was open. I wasn't sure what I was going to find. I found Peggy here.

How long could she have been like this? I mean . . . Has anyone seen her about?

I've only met her once before. That was two months ago. Out the front. Not like this. She was walking then. I've never been in her flat.

What's clear is that Peggy is trapped. The process probably began when she became tired or weak – perhaps through illness, perhaps self-neglect – and stopped performing the functions her body requires of her. As a solution, she has reduced her world to what she can reach: what goes into her body, what comes out of her body, and something to distract her brain. But now the supply of satsumas and yogurt has run out and the urine buckets are full, and she's sinking in a seeping amalgam of her own filth.

Can you get out of the chair, Peggy? Can you stand up and walk to the bathroom?

Yes.

Can you show us?

No.

Why not?

I'm watching.

What are you watching, Peggy?

No answer.

What are you going to eat?

No answer.

What day is it? Peggy? What day is it today?

No answer.

Do you have any family, Peggy?

No answer.

Any friends near by?

No answer.

Carers, Peggy? Do you have any carers?

No answer.

HEEP!

The smoke alarm.

Peggy?

Leave me be.

What do you think's going to happen if we leave you here?

Peggy's existence has come down to this moment. She is nothing but broken biology and crappy circumstance. An animal with no past, no context, no personality. Defenceless and dependent.

If she stays where she is, she will almost certainly die. This is how it happens. Not straightaway: her decline will be gradual at first. She's not struggling to breathe; her heart is not about to give up. But her legs have failed at their most basic function – to remove her from harm – and she'll contract an infection and the downward slope will steepen. Simply, she's in the pit and unable to climb out. She needs a helping hand.

No one else is coming. This is her chance. She has called out into the void and the rescuers are here. A funny-looking pair, but willing and able. She has the chance to be taken to a safe place, to be made clean and given a fresh start. Astonishingly, she wants to send us away.

Why do people refuse the assistance they clearly need? What rogue mutation of the psyche makes us so perverse?

It's an enduring paradox of this job that the patients who most need help are the ones who refuse it – while those with nothing wrong can't wait to get to A&E.

I'm sure there's an element of pride at work: often people are too stubborn to accept help. Many of us are also terrified of being an imposition – or, worse still, a waste of someone else's time. Perhaps Peggy doesn't realise how serious her situation is. Or perhaps she doesn't want to; denial can also be a powerful restraint.

If Peggy's mind is fixed on stoicism, it's a short journey from there to feeling ashamed of being ill; the work of a moment to find humiliation for admitting to dependence. Is Peggy's brain as trapped as her body?

In the cold analysis of black marks on a page, it seems unthinkable, almost offensive, to put the temporary shames that accompany physical incapacity before one's own safety, perhaps even life. But consider the reality of being dragged to hospital plastered in your own faeces, weak and defenceless, desperate to care for yourself but unable to perform even the most basic functions necessary to do so. There aren't many things worse than being trapped in your own private devastation – but one of them is surely having that devastation made public. Because even when we're ill or broken, even when we're entirely overwhelmed, we're more than just animals out of context in our broken biology.

Even with gloves on, the remote control looks toxic. I pick it up and press the red circle. The flat-screen kaleidoscope disappears. Silence. HEEP! I crouch down in front of the settee.

Here's what's going to happen, Peggy. We're going to stand either side of you and help you up. We're going to pop you in our chair and wrap you in this blanket. We'll take you out to the ambulance. It's early in the morning. There's no one around. No one's going to see you. We're going to run you up to the hospital. There won't be many people there, and we'll take you straight into a cubicle. They're going to get you clean and feed you and check you over. They're going to look after you, Peggy. They're going to help you get better.

Peggy shakes her head. She's clinging on. My colleague squats beside me.

I know you're scared, Peggy. I would be too. But when you heard your neighbour this morning, you called out for help. You knew something was wrong, didn't you? That's why you shouted out. And here we are. In a few hours' time, you'll feel so much better. I promise.

The neighbour puts his hand on her shoulder.

Come on, Peggy. Let them help you. Please?

There's a pause.

And then Peggy nods.

We move into position, one either side, and grasp the least soiled pieces of clothing we can find. We know the smell that's coming.

Ready, Peggy?

Peggy nods.

We take a deep breath.

11

II

My excursion into the ambulance world began on a whim. You could say I stumbled into this job. It was not my life's ambition to be a paramedic. I had no burning sense of purpose, no medical training, no experience as a carer. Hadn't done my time on patient transport or community response; never worked as a first aider in a marquee for St John's. I was an ingénue. A greenhorn. I had a passing notion of what the job entailed – car accidents, heart attacks, drunks – but had never arranged a ride-out to determine if my assumptions were correct. I was a nine-to-fiver in need of fresh air. A desk-jockey who thought fulfilment could be found in hardship. Call it the audacious life-change. Call it the impulsive allure of something new. Call it, perhaps, the reckless act of a creature without a plan.

BANG!

The eyes are wide. The head dipped. The nostrils flared in angry hoops.

BANG!

Shoulders low, arms pinned, torso straining against the cuffs.

BANG!

Threads of snot hang from his nose, cavorting to the rhythm of his rhino breaths.

BANG!

His forehead is friction-raw, a flattened strawberry, his teeth gritted, lips parted, jaw locked in a kind of spasm. The veins on his neck and his temples bulge. His face drips with sweat.

BANG!

He holds my gaze. Our faces are a metre apart.

BANG!

And every few seconds, he launches his body forward, and slams his skull against the screen.

BANG!

The reinforced Perspex rattles and shakes. The metal of the cage is beginning to warp. He steps back and snorts up the mucus and pushes out his chin and widens his eyes and snarls from deep in his throat.

BANG!

A breath, a snort, a tensing of the muscles, a head-butt.

BANG!

He's starting to sway. His shoulders roll from side to side. The police van takes a corner and he stumbles but regains his feet. He blinks and turns his head. Finally, now, is he going to stop?

BANG!

It's a performance. An exhibition. A petulant stride into the dark.

Bang!

A game of endurance. Holding a match until your fingers burn.

Bang!

Stabbing your hand with compass points.

Bang!

A game where a man is repeatedly smashing his head, as hard as he can, against a structure designed not to be breached.

Bang!

Until he wobbles and his eyes close. And his head goes back and his knees buckle. And he falls against the side of the van and collapses to the floor.

Bang!

At the age of six, all the boys at my school wanted to be lorry drivers or footballers. The girls played at ballerinas or teachers: that's just how it was. If you were a lorry driver you got to sit up high, and you could stop whenever you wanted and buy a Lion bar, and eat it behind the wheel, maybe with a can of Quattro. Or pull into Boss Hogs, the mysterious truck-stop café, for an all-day breakfast. This was in the eighties, when fibre was king and all food had to be brown by law: brown bread, brown rice, brown pasta, even brown cakes. To stop for sausage, egg and chips whenever you wanted was the stuff of adventure.

By the following year our ambitions had progressed to train driving – because someone found out that train drivers got to go faster than lorry drivers and they didn't have to worry about steering. There was a pretty sound logic there, although you'd have to plan ahead and bring the Lion bar in your packed lunch. The year after that the dream profession was astronaut (faster still), then zookeeper (school trip), policeman, fireman, stuntman. Never paramedic – or ambulance driver as we would have said then: let's be frank, it didn't seem tough enough; too much like being a nurse. I don't remember anyone saying they wanted to be an accountant or lawyer or civil servant. We hadn't been taught probability at that stage.

Careers classes at secondary school were a curious affair. The Head of Chemistry, a surprising selection perhaps, enthused at length on the successes of Sock Shop as a business model, and digressed extravagantly on the paradox of choice:

You kids are so lucky. So many choices. But, remember: to benefit from those choices you have to make *a choice. And . . . Bam! As soon as you've* made *a choice, all the other choices disappear . . .*

These eccentric homilies were followed by sessions of psychometric testing, designed to identify appropriate careers. The questionnaires set out ambiguous riddles and multiple-choice dilemmas –

Which of the following gives you the most satisfaction?

- *building a shelter for a wounded animal*
- *solving a mathematical puzzle in front of an audience*
- *organising a group of strangers to publish a community magazine*

– and used the results to assign future occupations to confused adolescents as if we were plugged into some sort of diagnostic supercomputer. Either the algorithm was skewed or my classmates were faking the answers, because almost everyone was advised to become a landscape gardener or a quantity surveyor – often, apparently, at the same time.

Of course, there were some kids who always knew what jobs they were going to do. Mostly these were the ones fated to follow in the footsteps of their parents, as if, without discussion, their entire futures were already planned out: the daughter of double-doctor parents who knew at thirteen she'd be taking three sciences and maths at A level; the son of a jeweller who was quick with figures and would leave school at sixteen to learn the family trade.

For most us, however, the idea of making plans for a future life of work was something to be avoided for as long as possible, because it acknowledged the prospect that one day, and for more than fifteen thousand subsequent days stretching out beyond the horizon, work was destined to become our master. We were busy with other things. We had CDs to copy onto C90 cassettes for friends, and elaborate cover designs to copy by hand, and since most albums were about 48 minutes long, there were tough choices to be made about which track to leave off so you could get one on each side. The music-less future was an inevitability to rebel against; if you submitted to it voluntarily, you were betraying your youth and your peers. It's a feeling that most of us, if we're honest, have never really left behind.

The call comes down as a twenty-five-year-old male. Unconscious, then a fit, then breathing problems. Then a fit again.

Reports are confused. It's at the police station, then out in the street. A message tells us police are on scene – patient 'kicking off'.

We pull up on a side street and find half a dozen officers kneeling on the pavement around a man on his side, a miscreant Gulliver, their arms extending to clamp various parts of his body in place. He wears combat trousers and heavy domed boots laced up his calves. He has cropped black hair and scars on his cheeks and a dark monobrow that dips in a V at the bridge of his nose. The skin of his face is pulled rigid across its bones, and the whites of his eyes are veined with tiny pink forks of fury. He is taut and tense, a trebuchet ready to launch.

You fucking cunts let go of me now or I'll stamp on every one of your fucking faces. I'll kick your fucking kneecaps until I snap them you cunts!

The tension in his muscles suggests he means what he says. He makes a sudden lunge to break free and his body writhes. The officers grip and hold and pin, but one of his legs gets loose and he kicks a female officer square in the chest with the sole of his boot. She's knocked backwards and rolls off her feet across the pavement, but gets up and dives back in and grabs his leg and pins it to the ground and again he is confined.

Heeeoooaaarrrggghhh!

He is a beast protesting capture. A rampaging fire fed fresh fuel yet to burn itself out. An overwhelmed force that will not surrender. A rage against the machine.

His body thwarted, the torrent of revolt is redirected

through his mouth. He stares at each officer in turn, demanding eye-contact, and shouting customised abuses:

You! Frankenstein! I'm gonna shit down your neck! And you, Fuckwit! You're gonna feel my boot up your arse til it knocks out your teeth!

The attacks are fired through the gaps in his broken Murray Mint teeth, spattered with saliva, adorned with obscenities, empowered and belittled and terrifying and absurd.

Apparently there was an altercation, some breaking of glass, then a fit. *An epileptic fit?* No one is sure: lots of angry shouting and thrashing about, is what the police have been told, which doesn't exactly sound like a seizure, but reports can't always be trusted. After more shouting, the police approached, which didn't improve the patient's mood. Told to calm down, lots of bluster and hostility, things went from bad to worse, with the patient stalking about and striking out. When the threat of violence got real they grabbed his arms. He had another fit, or episode of screaming, and eventually settled into his current state.

There's a woman with him, a timid girl in a large hood and thick glasses, clutching a case on wheels and a bag of belongings and staring at the wall. When I ask her what happened she looks at her feet and says she didn't see.

Does he have any medical conditions?

I don't know.

Does he take tablets?

No. Yes. I don't know what they're called. He's epileptic.

What's his name?

I only know his first name. Stephen.

What's Stephen's date of birth?

I don't know.

Okay. And you're his . . .?

Wife.

She turns her back and will say no more.

I take Stephen's wrist to feel his pulse. It's fast, like his breathing: he's clearly worked up, but the question is *why?* There are plenty of options. I put myself in the patient's eyeline, and speak as calmly as I can:

Stephen? Can you hear me, Stephen? Hello, mate. It's the ambulance. I'm sorry you're having a bad time. We're only here to help you. We want to make sure you're okay. Shall we see if we can calm things down? Make you a bit more comfortable? Will you let me check you over? Does that sound okay?

He looks me in the eye with a glare of pure, intimate hatred.

If you fucking touch me, gayboy, I'll kick the skull off the top of your neck and stamp on your fucking brains until they're part of the pavement.

Have you ever woken up and thought for a moment you were paralysed? There I was, in an air-conditioned office, with my right hand on a mouse and my left holding a mug of cold tea, and a sense that I may never be able to get out of this five-wheeled swivel chair because somehow it had become a part of me, or I of it. Perhaps I'd been daydreaming, or perhaps this was just where I lived now – with my legs tucked under the desk and a family pack of Kit Kats and a toothbrush in the bottom drawer? Was there a sleeping bag somewhere? A camp bed? A teasmade perhaps?

I had a screen full of unread emails in front of me, a list of tasks to cross off by the end of the day, a pile of project proposals to read through and report on – and a hazy dread in the back of my mind, that if I wasn't careful, I might fall asleep again and wake up in exactly the same position in forty years' time.

Stephen's going to A&E because there's nowhere else for him in this state. He won't sit in a chair or lie on a bed, and the officers can't hold him still in a moving vehicle. So he goes in the cage in the back of the police van. They assist him in and slam the doors. There's a seat but he's not interested in sitting down: he paces, as much as you can pace in a box the size of a shower cubicle. My place, with my gear, is in the other part of the back; on the safe side of the screen.

As soon as we pull away, the snorting and staring and head-butting begin.

BANG! . . . BANG! . . . BANG! . . . BANG!

It's a short journey, but long enough for some harm to be done. We've done everything we can to stop him. Now we put on the lights, warn the hospital we're coming. They are not going to be happy. I try to speak calmly, to persuade Stephen to stop hurting himself. But there's no halting this train. By the time he falls to the floor, I reckon he's smashed his head against the screen about twenty times.

Can you pull over please?

Problems?

He's collapsed.

Is he okay?

Not sure. Let's get him out.

We go to the back and they open the metal door, leaving the cage door closed for now.

Stephen? Stephen? You okay in there?

There's no response. They open the cage.

Stephen?

I take his wrist and feel a good, strong pulse. I open his eyes and shine a light. There's the faintest sensation of panic. But then Stephen shudders, does a double-take, and launches without missing a beat into a new volley of verbal abuse:

Get your fuckin hands away from me you filthy fuckin cunt! You! What the fuck you lookin' at? Eh?

We help Stephen back onto the seat, but he stands and starts kicking the inside of the box. We close the door again and jump back into the van and set off. The head-butts begin again:

Bang! . . . Bang! . . . Bang!

I never got spat on in my office job. Not pushed, punched or kicked – or threatened with physical violence. I wasn't often sworn at. Never had to work through the night, or at the weekend. All in all, it was pretty safe and sedate. And yet . . .

It wasn't that I hated my work. I just felt . . . shrivelled. Dehydrated. Compressed. Its day-to-day quirks kept my brain diverted, in the way that a good crossword keeps mental atrophy at bay but never takes aim at your deeper convictions. What was missing was any sense of necessity, of exhilaration, peril. Of being thrown in at the deep end. Or tested in ways that I couldn't anticipate in advance, or that would have any meaning beyond some numbers in a list of other numbers, or result in any kind of brokenness or repair, of shame or growth.

No doubt I was experiencing something familiar to us all: that soul-drain of vocational stunting; that yearning for a kick up the backside; or, as we all say when we complete the necessary forms, the desire for a new challenge. So, with a bloody-minded determination, I embarked on a project for which I was entirely unqualified, not to mention thoroughly ill-suited. Little did I know what I was letting myself in for.

III

The room is two metres by three: just big enough for a double bed and a cot. Plus a Moses basket and a car seat still in its plastic, and a stack of boxes and some bin bags bursting with clothes. And a chest of drawers with a TV on it. And five people. And a dog.

The curtains have been stretched to the middle of the window and pinned together with pegs, blocking out the sunlight. Save for a triangle of bright white duvet, the room is dark. I wait for my eyes to adjust.

What emerges from the gloom is a tableau. Poised in freeze-frame. Awaiting instruction. The woman who let me in hovers by the door. Her son, knelt on the one bare patch of floor, looks decidedly pasty, on the precipice of a faint, but I'm not here for him. His exhausted girlfriend, crying, laughing, flushed and sweating, naked except for a vest, her legs spread wide, leans back on her elbows in a marshland of saturated towels in the middle of the bed. And her daughter, less than five minutes old, pale, floppy, slathered in amniotic fluid and meconium and blood and draped loosely in a towel, lies in the space between her thighs.

Well, now. Congratulations!

Thanks.

Long before I contemplated a life in green, I'd received a warning that I failed to heed. A humbling personal insight that should have functioned as a *Keep Out!* sign, but instead set a ball rolling that's yet to stop.

It's funny how humiliation can act as a stimulant. Anyone who's endured an 'epic public fail' will know how the experience can spur you on. The initial impulse may be to take up residence in a nuclear bunker, but with time that thick cloud of regret morphs into a fiery determination to overcome, and before you know it, the juiciest shame has sown the seed of a minor victory.

I look around for somewhere to put my stuff. Like a tourist on a mystery holiday – or maybe a paramedic trying to pre-empt disaster – I've brought in everything I can carry.

For a moment all is quiet. Except there's also a dog. There's always a dog. Bouncing and yapping like a live-action metronome in the only space it can find – right between my legs. I speak to the new mum.

What's your name?

Rebecca.

Right, Rebecca. You've done really well. Boy or girl?

24

Girl.
Okay. Let's have a look at your little girl.

Ambulance crews have mixed feelings about maternities. To some these are the easiest calls in the world: the mum does the work and it's a simple case of catch, clean, clamp, cut, cuddle and congratulate. You get to participate in a significant moment in a family's life: smiles all round and a nice story to tell your friends. For others, births are messy, chaotic and stressful – but mainly messy – and if something goes wrong, you're a very long way from help. Midwives train long and hard to earn that unflappable demeanour, yet for ambulance staff, this is just one of an array of skills for which we profess a rudimentary but hopefully sufficient knowledge. I know of many crews who, happy to deal with major trauma, cardiac arrests and violent mental-health patients, will do everything they can to avoid having to open a maternity pack.

When I started out in the job, I think it's fair to say that nothing gave me a greater sense of dread than the idea of catching a new-born baby and taking responsibility for the first few minutes of its life. This was serious stuff, and I had form.

Today's maternity comes down to me mid-shift, in instalments, drip, drip, drip:

22 YR-OLD FEMALE, PREGNANT, IN LABOUR. CATEGORY 2.

I'm four miles away, alone in a fast-response car. I set off on lights and sirens, but it sounds pretty innocuous so far. I get trapped at a junction and the screen beeps. Next instalment:

WATERS BROKEN

Then:

URGE TO PUSH

You can almost feel the tension rising down the line. I stuff a handful of gloves in my pocket and mentally check the equipment I'll need. It's difficult to tell but I'm inclined to caution. Urge to push I've heard before: I still have my doubts until I see for myself.

Then, a minute later:

BABY OUT. CATEGORY I.

I'm two miles away. I'll be first there, but there should be an ambulance right behind. A further beep:

BABY FLOPPY. DIFFICULTY BREATHING

Then a message from Control:

NO AMBULANCE TO SEND. PLEASE PROVIDE UPDATE

Rough translation: *You're on your own.*

The instinctive reaction is foot to the floor. Diesel. Sirens. Boldness. Speed. Zooming through traffic because every second counts. But instinct's folly and craves restraint; the other view prevails. Composure. Clarity. Progress, not haste. Enhanced velocity but no extra risk.

I picture the swan. Method, method. Slow, deep breaths. Serenity above the eyeline. I decide what I'll take in, plan what I'll do first. Take a moment to assess. Keep everything simple. There'll be no setting off for hospital, so I'll treat what I can treat.

At least, that's the idea.

The first thing I do is turn around and walk out of the room. I drop all my bags in the hall, then come back in with what I need now: the maternity pack and oxygen bag.

Can you put the dog away, please?

He won't be happy.

He'll get over it.

The dog tries to dart under the bed, but the new grand-mother's in no mood for games. She seizes the collar and slides it yelping from the room on the laminate. I step past the new dad.

Feeling a bit rough?

I think he's overwhelmed.

Your girlfriend's done all the work!

I rip open the maternity pack.

I'm only joking, mate. It's a shock, isn't it? Why don't you climb up on the bed? Make a bit of space there. Have a lie down.

The new dad clambers onto the bed like he's summiting Everest and leans against the wall. His face is grey.

Right, let's have a little look at baby. You know what time she came out?

I take baby from Mum and lie her on the towel.

Five minutes ago?

She's still attached so can't come far: it's all very familiar at moments like this. I begin drying baby.

Have you got a name?

27

Not yet.

Baby's breathing but I'm yet to hear a cry. I start with the head and face, rubbing vigorously, wiping away the gunge of the recent ordeal, then down to the chest and back, mopping up the glistening moisture, flipping the towel to find dry patches for the buttocks and limbs, stimulating the body to respond. I'd be a lot happier if I heard a cry.

My radio buzzes:

General broadcast, general broadcast, ambulance required, still holding a BBA, FRU on scene, any ambulances please make themselves available.

This is me. BBA: born before arrival. No one's coming just yet.

I'm a little concerned but I don't want the parents to see. Mum looks exhausted and Dad's pale as a sheet. A dose of panic might finish him off. At the moment I have two patients. I don't want a third.

Baby's colour isn't great and her body is still floppy. These are things that should improve when she's properly oxygenated. What this little girl needs is to scream: the traumatised shriek of the new-born; the vigorous complaint of someone thrown out of paradise and dumped in a puddle. The squeal that pushes the fluid from the lungs and fills them with air. So far she hasn't made a sound.

Anyone who's ever felt surplus to requirements will understand the plight of the expectant father when the day of reckoning arrives. The term *spare part* has never been so apt. Child-bearing is enough of a mystery to the male mind at the best of times, but it's only once the race towards a messy conclusion is under way that the male participant, until now convinced he is central to what's occurring, becomes suddenly aware of his own irrelevance. In the plainest terms, what can he contribute? His biology is nine months out of date. He has no skills to offer. The escalating agony of his partner? He is powerless to change this. The impending arrival of his child? This will happen with or without his involvement. Never has a human being been so heavily invested in a situation he can do so little to affect.

This is the reality that Rebecca's boyfriend, James, is currently facing, and he appears to be deep in thought on the subject. It's possible he's contemplating the irony that fathering a child should be the event in life that makes one feel most impotent. Or perhaps he's just finding the whole thing a bit grim.

On the sidelines of labour, the diligent male is torn between competing impulses. He wants to support his partner – to contribute, to encourage, to be a good guy – but he's out of his comfort zone and terrified of saying or doing the wrong thing. He can't experience the agony – but perhaps he can sympathise?

Do you want some water?

No! No!

She pushes it away.

Are the contractions getting worse?

Of course they're getting worse!

Maybe they'll get better soon . . .?

I don't want them to get better! I want them to get worse! That's the whole point. Didn't you read the book?

Actually, no, he skipped that chapter. It was making him feel ill.

Water!

He puts the cup to her lips.

Give me your hand!

He holds out his hand and she grips it, grimaces – another contraction. She digs in her nails and squeezes, then squeezes some more. He's just happy to be of use.

The alternative strategy, much favoured by tactful males of previous generations, is to make oneself scarce. This is also known as running away. On the 'out of sight, out of mind' principle, the benefits are clear, but they have their perils. By absenting himself without leave, the new father risks a life-long reputation as a deserter from the frontline.

However, there is a third way. In this scenario, the culpable male is able to be both present and absent at the same time; at once notionally supportive and yet utterly, blissfully useless. How can this be so? The new dad achieves this with a surprisingly popular tactic: fainting.

This is the method Rebecca's boyfriend, James, seems to have adopted. In fact, James hasn't gone the whole hog and passed out on the floor, but he has found refuge in a state of what we might call gentle infirmity. Whether James would rather be a fainter than a deserter is unclear. Either way, it's a good job his mother was on scene to pick up the slack.

Did she cry when she came out?
No.

Has she cried since?

No. Is that bad?

It's okay. We might just need to help her.

Is something wrong?

I'm going to cut the cord, okay?

I attach three plastic clamps: one each side plus one for luck. It's jelly-smooth, rope-tough, spiralled and bulging like a sea creature. I use the curved scissors to snip, snip, keeping two clamps on baby's side. I wrap her in a dry towel and lie her back on the bed, then duck out of the room for the suction unit. I've spotted some yellow-brown bubbles around her nostrils when she breathes: she may have taken in some meconium during the delivery. Using a tiny plastic tube, I remove the traces from the mouth and nostrils.

How you feeling, Mum?

Okay.

She's starting to look worried.

Not dizzy?

No.

Still contracting?

No, it's stopped. Is she okay?

Yep, I just want to check her a bit more.

It looks like something's wrong?

I unwrap my stethoscope and listen to baby's chest: I can hear the heartbeat, see the chest moving, but I'm still unhappy with baby's colour, and the fact she's limp – and quiet. I take the small bag-valve mask from its packet and place the tiniest mask on the baby's face – little bigger than a rubber thimble.

Don't be alarmed, Mum. She's breathing. I just want to help her out.

Is she okay?

This can be quite common. It's just a bit of assistance.

I lay the steth on baby's chest and hold the mask in place. I listen for the breathing and squeeze the bag to push air into the lungs. I tell myself to be gentle – the lungs are tiny, and my arms are charged with enthusiasm. It's barely a pinch of the bag, and the chest expands.

I do this for half a minute. It's a delicate interlude of apparent composure. But looks can be deceptive. As I watch the chest, squeezing gently on the bag, a dozen thoughts rush into my brain. Is Mum bleeding? I haven't checked her yet. Is baby getting cold? But it's warm in here. Does she have meconium in her lungs? How worried are the parents? Is Dad about to pass out? Is there anything I'm missing? There must be something I'm missing. What's the plan if baby doesn't perk up? If I was in a maternity unit I could push the big red button on the wall and a team of midwives and obstetricians would appear. Here the only button to press is on my radio, and help is still miles away. Is backup even coming?

And, in the end, the central question: am I doing this right?

Perhaps it's James's plight that's making me doubt myself. The new father's predicament, close to horizontal and unable to participate in this momentous event, is a bit too familiar for my liking. It takes me back to the birth of my first child, my own 'epic fail', when I stood by and cheer-led, and stood by and proffered glucose tablets, and stood by and fetched, and stood by a little bit longer while things got tenser and more people appeared, until the crucial moment came and I became abruptly aware that standing by was something I wasn't able to do any more. As my son made his first appearance, the heat flushed upwards through my body and the solid world took on a fluid quality and began to shift in front of me, and I turned and spotted a well-placed chair and made a beeline for it just in time.

It could be argued that the inability to stay upright at moments of clinical drama should not point towards a career in emergency medicine. Indeed, some might say that an experience like this ought to be taken as an injunction against such a path. What if it were to happen again? Imagine the consequences if, at a crucial moment in the throes of someone's crisis, I came over woozy and took the horizontal path . . .

Yet isn't it human nature to put ourselves to the test? It may have been an instinctive decision, but I soon became aware of its implications. I was forced to befriend my flaws and give them accommodation: my lack of experience, my apprehension, my vague phobia of red sticky fluids. They loomed large in my thinking as I made the switch. They accompanied me into my training and pursued me out onto the road. If I had lamented the absence of struggle, of antagonism, then now I had found it: that dread of a repeat performance in an arena where the safety nets would be in short supply. I had volunteered for a process of compensation; to build a scaffold of preparation around my embarrassing secret, in the restless hope that with time it would come to bear the weight itself. I was far from sure.

As I kneel over this new-born, several years later, gently

squeezing oxygen into her lungs, I feel like I've come a long way, and no distance at all. The friendly terror endures, but I'm neither the first nor the last to experience that. It's all in the context. A different role, a different setting. A memory to keep complacency at bay. All those unique and everyday details – the lack of space, the heat, the mess, the medical equipment that I've brought inside; the mum exhausted and desperate for reassurance, the father slumped against the wall, the eager grandma, the barking dog; and especially the tiny, helpless child – are not just the minor challenges of an assignment in the real world, they're also the protective markers of distance that keep the mind on the job. There'd be no place for any other response. The swan, the swan. Process. Calm.

I lift off the mask and watch the breathing again. Baby's colour is better; her muscles are flinching and relaxing. I push gently in the centre of the chest: the skin goes white momentarily, then flushes back to a deep pink. She gasps a deep breath and there's a frozen moment. Her limbs shudder and wince; then she cries out.

It's a flat rubbery wail that comes out weakly at first but then builds in strength. Another gasp, the chest expanding, then the same again, but louder: *Waaa-aaah! Waaa-aaaah!* Suddenly she has a miniature siren all of her own. It's the most pitiful, soothing and welcome sound in the world.

Her skin blooms with colour, and her muscles seem to be energised with outrage at her new situation. A crimson hue that shouts: *How dare you?*

After the cry she takes several rapid breaths, then settles into a more plaintive whimper. I listen to her heart: it's racing happily, too fast to count. I rewrap her in the towel, scoop her up and pass her to Mum, who holds her to her chest, and the whimpering subsides.

I put my hands behind my back, so the parents won't see them shake.

IV

It's the kind of night you wouldn't go out in unless you had to. Cold. Dark. Windy. Wet. Sunday evening: the soggy remnant of the weekend. The rain batters the pavements, stirring up the encrusted grime and sending cascades of yeasty water along the gutters. Leaves have been blown into dunes of autumnal slush and bags of litter have been shredded by foxes, their contents strewn across the pavements and roads.

Late-night hunter-gatherers scurry out of corner shops clutching milk and bread, dodging puddles on the way to cars with hazards blinking across the reflective glaze. In the doorways of chicken shops, groups of boys in hoods stare at the screens of their phones. Exhausted shift-workers huddle under bus shelters. And calmly, deliberately, oblivious to the deluge, bedraggled revellers stumble merrily home.

It's the fourth of four nights and the fatigue's starting to hit. I'm a week into my new existence and yet to master daytime sleep. Not quite fresh-faced and bright-eyed, then, but certainly raw and not a little petrified of the thousand things that could go wrong. The meal-deal lunch and that

Friday feeling are things of the past: I've cashed them in to spend my weekends and nights on the bejewelled urban streets, in a thousand aromatic bedsits, and queueing in an assortment of convivial A&Es, all in the name of going home with a warm sensation in my chest – probably the heartburn from eating dirty chicken at three a.m.

Everything in this new world is unfamiliar and unnerving: the jargon, the equipment, the etiquette, the access codes. Using the phonetic alphabet on the radio; detaching the suction unit from the ambulance wall; acknowledging police cars when you're at work but never in your own car, or realising at the last moment and nonchalantly running your hand through your hair instead. There's a way of folding the blanket around the patient so it doesn't get caught in the wheels of the chair, and a way of folding the chair so you don't trap your fingers, and a way of deploying the tail-lift so the bed doesn't go flying, patient and all, off the end, and there's a different way of booking in at every hospital, and a different code to get in in the first place, and a different place to stand as you wait for the nurse to acknowledge your existence, and sometimes even a line you mustn't cross, which is hard to believe but seems to be a thing, like lining up in the playground, and there's somewhere to put your dirty sheet and somewhere else to get a clean one in return, and maybe a blanket, but there are some hospitals that won't let you take a blanket, as if you're going to sell it on eBay rather than bring it back in an hour's time, and there are some that won't let you have a sheet, even though you just brought one in, and there are some places you can get a cup of tea, some where you can nip into reception to use the kettle, or if you know the nurse maybe the staff room, but heaven forbid you should get any of this wrong, because then it will be abundantly clear that you're a novice and there's no one lower than that.

I've been told about a hundred times: the one thing I must do is get us off on time – otherwise my name will go round the mess room quicker than the latest rumours about that crew that got suspended somewhere out east. Before I press the green button that makes us available, I ask:

You okay if I go green?

You do whatever you want, geeze. As long as you get me off on time . . .

It's a lottery. While we're with a patient, we're untouch-able. But once that job's finished, we offer up for the next encounter. At any given time, the service is holding a backlog of calls, across a range of priorities. The details have been taken, the addresses confirmed and the symptoms fed into the triage algorithm. You hit that button and you don't know which of them is going to land in your lap:

Happy to do another?

You're in charge. But whatever you do, don't get me off late. Understand?

It's just timing and geography. When a job's waiting in the system, the computer will dispatch the nearest available crew. But there's always the prospect of being cancelled off an amber for a red:

Ready to go available?

Born ready, mate. But you need to make this one last. I can't be off late tonight, I got plans . . .

A ten-second delay in hitting that button might be the difference between a stabbed torso and a stubbed toe.

Standard procedure when everything's fresh is to assume the worst at all times: all chest pains will be heart attacks; any mention of haemorrhage will mean a slaughterhouse of claret sprayed across the floor and walls; and difficulty breathing will be someone gasping their last. Of course, this is rarely the case, as I'm starting to find out. But with an absence of experiential data to fall back on, the tendency is to believe whatever appears on the dispatch screen. So when, halfway through the shift, a call comes down stating

38-YR-OLD MALE

POSSIBLE COLLAPSE BEHIND LOCKED DOORS

in my brain, at least, it's all systems go. My crewmate for the night, who's done many years and never has trouble finding a sheet, and even a blanket, is less impressed.

This call is a flirt. A swindle, a tease. The locked door is the perennial MacGuffin that fires the imagination, and the vagueness of the description – that *possible* collapse – suggests shady misadventures in hidden rooms. What would keep a thirty-eight-year-old from getting to the door? A broken ankle? A stroke? Drugs? Drink? A really deep sleep? Or even, of course, the lack of a pulse. This job could be anything from a week-dead corpse to a man who's popped to the off-licence without his phone.

The address is given as a flat on the High Road, but that's a line of shops so it's going to be accessed from the back. We turn down the side-street and pull up beside a gate ripped off its hinges. Behind the gate stretches an unlit alleyway along the back of the shops and takeaways. It's overgrown with bushes and debris and the obligatory shopping trolley. This is where the businesses keep their bins, and passers-by toss their half-eaten takeaways, and the local rats go for a week's all-inclusive, and who knows what else occurs. It's a place you'd be disinclined to venture if you weren't in uniform – yet this is someone's garden path.

I'm eager to get in there and find out what's going on. I've yet to experience a really nasty job, and I sense that this one has potential. It's a kind of burden, the desire to pop the cherry and get that first cardiac arrest or decent trauma under your belt – like the club's new signing who wants to hit the back of the net before it becomes an issue. My crewmate, however, seems in less of a rush.

Don't get too excited. It's gonna be a pile of crap.

You never know.

Believe me. I can tell.

He takes his time parking so that the side light illuminates the alleyway, then grabs the torch as well. He moves without any sense of haste. I take the bags and we push on into the gloom. The horizontal strands of a dozen spider-webs attach themselves to our faces. Something scurries further into the dark. Along one side of the alley, the unpainted fire doors are scrawled with numbers, and makeshift letterboxes have been attached to the fence with wire. At the address we want, the narrow passage opens into a tiny yard, and beside a large doorway there's an intercom with four unlabelled buzzers.

My radio vibrates every time the job updates, which only

puts me more on edge. This is it, I can feel it. I'm going to do some real work. But the messages themselves are little help: more information making things less clear. The caller isn't the patient and isn't on scene: it's unclear who or where they are. They're sure the patient is in the flat, and adamant he can't get to the door. But they won't say why. The police have been dispatched.

We've tried all the buzzers to no effect. We've called through the letterbox, banged on the window. We've asked Control for more details, but it's like Chinese whispers: I speak to a dispatcher in another part of town, so they can call the origin, a third party at a second location, for them to try to contact the patient – who, dead or alive, indisposed or asleep, is probably just a few feet away from where I stand. They say the patient's stopped answering his phone. Last contact an hour ago. All they'll say is he can't get up.

The police arrive with the Enforcer, a solid metal cylinder with handles. It targets the point where the lock meets the frame and often knocks out part of the structure, but it won't work on the external door here because the hinges are reversed. The officer uses a crowbar instead, attacking the door with relish. It's an incredibly noisy process, and it destroys a section of the door and a large part of the frame. You'd have to be very unwell to let someone do this much damage to your front door without getting up to protest.

There's no response from any of the flats: everything points to a real emergency inside.

By now we've been given a flat number, and we bang on the second door. There's a murmur from inside. The patient's alive. But still not coming to let us in. Could he be trapped under a wardrobe? Is his heart about to give up? I shout through the letterbox – tell the patient we've had to break one door to get this far, and we'll have to do the same again if he can't get up. All I get in response is a dull murmur.

This time the Enforcer does its job, and the heavy door flies back on its hinges, with part of the frame flying across the room. I call out and go in. The hallway is dark, the light has no bulb: this, I'm discovering, is a common theme. I follow the murmur to a small room filled with big furniture: a bed on one side, a sofa on the other, with just a two-foot gap in between. For my selfish mind and its desire to get established, this is the moment of truth. I'm partly dreading and partly hoping that I'll find something really grim.

In the two-foot gap, on his back, groaning and wincing, beating his fists on the floor, lies a thirty-eight-year-old man. I may be a rookie but even I can see: this man is not trapped, and he also isn't dying. What he is, is lying on the floor. Am I disappointed? A little, yes, I have to admit. Am I relieved? On his behalf, yes, naturally, that too.

Pain is horrible, of course. We all know that; we've all experienced pain and we've all made our feelings on the subject abundantly clear. But it's not always a disaster. Being in pain entails awareness; *conveying* that pain requires effort. People who are really unwell – critically unwell – rarely make a lot of noise or writhe around because their bodies are too busy being ill.

When he's asked what's wrong, the patient covers his eyes

with one hand and reaches the other round to his lower back and sobs.

You have back pain?

He nods.

When did the pain start?

He shakes his head.

You don't know? Today?

He groans and shakes his head again.

What day then?

The patient lifts his hand and slowly extends three fingers.

Three days ago? Thursday?

He nods.

Did you have an accident? Car accident?

He shakes his head.

Did you fall?

He shakes his head.

Did you bang your back on something?

He shakes his head.

Have you been here since Thursday?

He shakes his head.

Why can't you speak? Sir? What's wrong with your voice?

The patient opens his mouth and moves his lips without uttering any sound. I lean in closer.

Sorry, sir. Try that again. A bit louder.

The patient gulps. He licks his lips as if he's just emerged from the desert. He whispers:

Too . . . much . . . pain.

Okay. We can get you some gas and air for the pain.

I glance at my crewmate; he shrugs and turns to go.

It's really good stuff, it's going to help. Let me just do a few quick checks. But just tell me, what were you doing when the pain started? Were you at work?

The patient shakes his head, and pats the seat of the sofa that's beside him.

You were sat on the sofa?

The patient shakes his head again. He extends his arm flat.

You were lying on the sofa?

The patient nods. No one told me charades was going to be such a big part of this job.

While the police are arranging for the two broken doors to be secured (they'll need to be fixed later, at considerable cost), and my crewmate fetches the pain relief, I start running a few checks: blood pressure, pulse, oxygen levels, temperature. Then the patient's phone rings.

It's on the bed beside the patient, no more than a foot from his hand. He hasn't reported any problems with his arms, but now he signals that he needs the phone to be passed to him. I have to climb over him to get to the phone. I hold it out, but he doesn't take it; he leaves it in my hand and swipes the screen with his finger. If I was concerned he was unable to speak, I can fret no more: he thunders a greeting at whoever's just given him a call. He seems to have found his voice.

One of the assumptions about ambulance work is that everyone doing the job must be really *lovely*. Gentle. Kind. Sympathetic to all. Impervious to abuse. Immune to the smell of vomit. Tolerant of family members who've jumped to the worst of conclusions. Placid in the face of advice from helpful bystanders who once did a first-aid course. Offering a supportive elbow and a cheeky remark to the old ladies; putting terrified kids at their ease with soothing tones and up-to-date cultural references. Real-world Samaritans in green combats who never let a hard word cross their lips or a mean thought fester in their minds.

The natural correlative to this theory is that the work itself provides its own reward. That people doing the job get a warm, gooey feeling from all the times they know they've helped others, and this keeps them *nice*. One day you might save someone's life! Another you might deliver a baby! Or take away someone's pain, or stop them being scared. If you happen to get abused or sworn at from time to time, if you kneel in someone's urine or get coughed on or spat at, this is all just part of the feedback system – unpleasant, maybe, but part of the deal. What more could anyone want?

'You must find your job so rewarding,' people say.

'Hmmm . . . Sometimes,' comes the tentative reply.

The rest of this encounter plays out in a haze of what you might call showmanship. I may only be a week in, but already I'm learning how to play the part: sing-song sympathy wrapped around a sceptical resolve. The patient performs with a great deal of passion but also a touch of inconsistency. He hollers, he cries, he winces, he gulps on the gas. He says it's not helping, but won't let it go. We help him up, and since he's adamant he needs hospital, we take him in. I'm in no doubt he's in pain, but it's clear he's done very little in the way of self-care.

On a chest of drawers not two metres from where he lies shouting at his phone, I find a form from an A&E department on the other side of town, dated two days earlier and scrawled '*Lower Back Pain*', along with two packs of strong painkillers: naproxen and tramadol, real humdingers. One pack has one tablet missing; the other is full. All the pieces of the jigsaw are there.

He shows no concern for the two broken doors as we convey him to the local A&E. Possibly he doesn't connect their current state with his actions. I feel vaguely indignant on someone's behalf, but I'm not quite sure whose. His flatmates, his landlord? His worried friend at the other end of the phone? The NHS at large? Those faceless financiers, the payers of tax?

For myself, I've been duped by my own impatience and a simple dramaturgical trick. I won't be ticking anything as spicy as cardiac arrest off my list today; I'll have to wait for my first clear shot on goal.

My crewmate hands me a cup of tea when we're back in the truck; I've no idea where he found it at this time of night. We have six minutes to drink it, then it's time to go green.

You okay to do another?

Ready when you are. So long as you get me off on time.

V

I pull up in the dead of night, but the scene is already buzzing
with activity. Flashing blue lights and vigorous parking; steel-
toed boots striding about with purpose. Uniforms nodding
to each other, shaved heads conferring in clipped exchanges.
There's a couple of fire trucks, a handful of police vehicles,
and some transport responders all looking busy. But there's
no ambulance proper yet, so they're stuck with me in the
first-response car – a lettuce leaf at a barbecue.

The surrounding streets are quiet. In the early hours of
Monday morning, the rational world is tucked up under its
duvet. Where I stop there's no sign of the incident. The call's
come down as a fall from height, but there's no body sprawled
on the pavement, no victim bent double clutching a bloody
face. The address was given as a tanning salon – but who goes
on a sunbed at one in the morning? Now I'm here it seems
to be a Cash Converters – are all these people here for a stolen
Xbox?

*It's round the back and down the stairs. You want a hand with
your gear?*

Thanks. In a basement?
A bit further down than that. What's your call-sign?
I tell him.
You got a torch?
In here somewhere.
Feeling fit?
Is it far?
It's a warren. Follow me. And watch your step.

I take everything I might need and follow the officer along an unlit alley between the buildings. Past the industrial bins, through some tall metal gates topped with barbed wire, into a small service yard and through a concealed doorway. We're at the top of a metal staircase which spirals down into the darkness. Torchlight bounces below as other figures descend.

What is this place?
Who knows?

Down, down, round, round we follow, plodding carefully: clunk, clunk, clunk ring our boots on the gridded steps. I've come down at least five storeys by the time I reach the bottom and step into a kind of industrial labyrinth. The air down here is warm and fetid and tastes of soot, as if I've stumbled across a nineteenth-century mine. There are tunnels behind locked gates, oversized pipes and cables, sets of steps leading off in all directions. And on the walls a thick, dark grime. I'm on a mystery tour of the world beneath the streets.

I continue along the passageway, and then one of the walls abruptly disappears. I find myself surveying a giant cavern. The room opens out below and above and abroad to both sides. It could be the backstage area of an underground theatre; more likely it's a disused storage room with some industrial purpose, perhaps a thing of the past. It's too dark in here to see the ceiling or the walls, but in the murky gloom cast by a couple of spotlights, I can make out a scaffold tower. Beyond the tower, several torches point down into a crater in the floor.

I'm guessing that's where our patient is?
Apparently.

The main floor area is strewn with rubble and rubbish, and accessed via a wooden step ladder propped against the ledge I'm standing on. I lower my equipment, then follow it down, walking gingerly over to the hole in the floor.

When I reach the edge of the pit I can see why I'm here.

The depth of the hollow is unclear, because it contains a haphazard selection of building debris: poles and bars protruding at chaotic angles, sections of moulded steel, various broken and rusting corrugated shards. And on top of this wreckage, sort of nestled within it, about a metre down, neither screaming nor shouting, lies a man on his back in overalls and a football shirt.

He's breathing and conscious and doesn't appear to be impaled. He has injuries certainly, as yet unknown. At first glance, he's a tough man silently smothering his pain. His workmates scurry around, clearing the way, holding lights, trying to help. This was not how their night was supposed to pan out.

Did you see what happened?
One minute he was on the platform. Next thing I heard a crash.
This is how he landed?

We haven't moved him.
Well done. What's his name?
Gary.
Which platform was Gary on?
The top one.

I look back up at the scaffold and make a rough estimate: about a ten-metre drop. High likelihood of significant injury. Life-threatening? Perhaps. Serious spinal injury? Quite possibly. The contents of the pit look like the discard pile from a torture exhibition at the Tower of London; who knows what he's landed on? Perhaps it cushioned his fall. More likely, a protruding beam has performed some localised mutilation, maybe ruptured an organ. I need to get down there and investigate. It's a cat's cradle of steel and iron, but I can just about see where to put my feet.

There are many ways to find out you're unprepared. You might get gently pulled aside: *I'm not letting you go out like that.* Someone might halt you in your tracks: *Don't step in that!* A door might politely close in your face: *I'm afraid you've been unsuccessful at this stage.* Or you might get your own sense of foreboding and abort and turn back.

But, of course, you might only realise how ill-equipped you are once it's too late: when, one Sunday evening, you fall into a pit full of rubble from a great height in the dark. Or, perhaps, when you experience your debut anxiety attack in a corporate hospitality suite full of people on the first day of your new job as a trainee paramedic . . .

Having narrowly avoided a tête-à-tête with the floor of

the delivery room a couple of years earlier, and concluded that a new career involving blood, stress and medical trauma was the only sensible response, I'd applied to the ambulance service as something of an experiment. I never thought I'd get in; I assumed I would be found out along the way and that would be that. But no: at each stage I passed the assessments and was allowed through another gate, and the process took on a momentum of its own. By the time I'd stopped to consider if this jaunt was the height of folly, I was on my induction with other new recruits, listening to a lecture on basic life support in a stifling room devoid of natural light. It was only at this point that my temperamental shortcomings chose to make themselves apparent – in a physical manifestation that threatened to derail my new project before it had even begun.

Hello, Gary. How you doing, buddy?

I've been better.

He takes tiny wincing breaths.

Gary, we're going to get you out. But I need to check you over. Try not to move.

Not much danger of that.

I balance my feet amid the junk: one on a kind of girder, the other on a mesh panel. I bounce gently to see if either shifts. They hold firm for now. Everything I touch, my gloves come back black.

Let me feel your wrist. You fell from the top?

Well I didn't jump . . .

Glad to hear it. Did you hit your head?

Don't think so.

Were you knocked out?

Too much pain for that.

I run my hands over Gary's skull.

Were you wearing a helmet?

He shakes his head.

Try not to move. Keep your head still. Any pain when I touch?

In my arm. And my back.

Your head?

No.

Here on your neck?

No.

Where on your back?

Down there.

Gary uses his left hand to point to the bottom of his ribs. He can't use his right because that arm is floppy – and swollen and twisted. A fractured humerus, I guess.

I'm going to give you some oxygen, okay?

There's nowhere to put anything. I balance the cylinder on a crate, hoping it won't slip down a gap and disappear. I connect the mask and slide it over Gary's face.

We'll get you something for the pain really soon.

I put my hands across Gary's chest.

Take a deep breath.

I can't.

Too painful?

He nods. As he breathes, his chest lifts and expands. The left side is taut, round, a rigid balloon, but the right feels concave, like a car door that's been driven into.

I need to listen to your chest. I'm going to have to cut your shirt.
Do you have to?
Afraid so. Sorry.
Not a football fan?
Not really.
Lucky you.

As I balance on the girders, assessing and treating what I can on an unsteady footing, it occurs to me that this is what my friends think I do all the time. Critical trauma in strange locations. Life-threatening emergencies on shifting ground. The biro in the trachea. The tourniquet on the side of the road. Basically, re-enacting episodes of *Casualty*. This sort of thing should be a paramedic's bread and butter. In fact it's closer to a whole dressed lobster: a meal you've heard of, and read about, and maybe even eaten once or twice – but one that takes a bit of concentration if you're not going to spill the sauce down your shirt with everyone watching. At times like this, I'm not so much doing my job as doing an excellent imitation of the person whose job I'm looking after until they get back from wherever they went.

Gary's plight has layers. It's not a clinical crisis in isolation; there are logistical obstacles as well. His body's in a pretty bad place, yes, but it's also in a pretty bad *place*. And right now the complications of his situation are zipping around my head like tiny little yelps of torment. Paper aeroplanes with messages scrawled across the wings, that glide in front of me then drop to the floor. It's as if my brain is heckling itself: *Get a grip. Come on, buddy. Do what needs to be done.*

I'm sure there are people who never doubt themselves. And I'm sure there are others who just know how to fake it. But, for me, jobs like this take me back to that very first day in the conference centre, several years before, and my own impending plunge into a pit. It was the watershed moment. There was no going forward or back.

I became hot and dizzy, and the room felt airless and began to turn. I started shifting in my seat, light-headed and fidgety and desperate to silence the white noise in my head. I was sure I must be attracting attention, but tried to project an outward image of calm. I could tell my face was clammy, and I wanted to lean over and put my head between my knees – but this would have been like raising my hand and calling out, 'I'm sorry, I've made a massive mistake,' and leaving there and then. I had too much invested for that. Could I slip out of the room without making a scene? I'd do anything for a mouthful of fresh air. A sip of water. No, I'd have to stay. But what would happen if I actually passed out? I would end up a kind of legend; a preposterous real-life cautionary tale.

This is the feeling that revisits me now. Not the threat of collapse or failure, but the deafening roar of timidity. A cacophony of pessimists inside my head, telling me Gary would be better off with someone else. The whispering voices that call me impostor. The bickering experts that are as helpful as silence when you're trying to make a plan.

You hanging in there, Gary?

Yep.

I'm gonna put a needle in your arm. Give you something for the pain. You might feel a little scratch.

I doubt it.

I balance my cannula roll across two metal bars, tie a glove around Gary's left arm as a tourniquet, wipe the skin, then slide the needle into the vein. I pull the glove away, retract the needle and tape the cannula in place, then push some salty water into the vein.

I need to check your blood pressure, Gary. This is going to squeeze your arm.

The clamorous pessimists are getting impatient: *Why are we farting around with pain relief? Gary has multiple fractures, several in his chest, plus some likely organ damage and the potential for a spinal injury. We need to get him out.*

But there's another voice, a calm opponent with a contrasting view: *Gary's breathing, awake and calm; he's able to speak and not losing large quantities of blood. He's even making the odd joke, which is a good sign. And so far his body's coping pretty well.*

Yes, but he's thirty metres underground. Down a spiral staircase. In a pit filled with metal junk. Unable to move. In the dark. One by one, the pessimists have laid down their cards.

The optimist, however, is clear and composed: *None of these problems is insurmountable. Let's take things in a logical order. Gary's surrounded by people who are here to help.*

Above me, the trauma doctor arrives: I give him a brief handover before he lowers himself into the pit to make some more assessments himself.

It looks like Gary's sustained a 'flail chest', where a portion of his ribs has detached from the main structure – hence the lack of expansion on that side. The space between his ribs and lungs may be filling with air, or blood, and gradually restricting his ability to breathe. It's only one of several problems, none of which can be fixed here. At the moment the doctor's happy Gary's stable. But things can always change.

The hurdle is the location. Gary's on oxygen and has had some morphine, but his injuries require a swift journey to a trauma hospital for definitive care. The ace up the pessimists' sleeve is the fact that Gary, in spite of his breathing problem, needs to be kept as still as possible, and standing between him and that swift journey are a shipment of loose metal, a seven-foot climb up a wooden ladder and a hundred-plus steps up a spiral staircase.

But here the optimist comes into his own.

First the trauma doctor decides that he doesn't need to intervene any further with the breathing, and the extrication can proceed calmly, with due protective caution for Gary's neck and back. Right on time, a crew brings the relevant gear down the spiral stairs.

Second, one of the site managers announces that if we can get Gary out of the pit and lift him onto the wooden ledge, then down another flight of stairs, we can carry him along a tunnel to another site with an industrial lift half a mile up the road.

Did you say half a mile?

It's that or the spiral stairs.

It looks like the shaved heads on standby will be required . . .

We wrap Gary up like a Fabergé egg and slide a board underneath. The morphine's working: he's more relaxed. We lift him from the crater and place him in a bucket stretcher I've never seen before. There's a dispute about how to get him up to the ledge, but the muscles from the fire brigade end the discussion by raising him to head height and sliding him on: it takes three seconds.

With bearers on each side, Gary is lifted to waist height and carried down the stairs to the tunnel. The bearers climb down into the trench and the stretcher is slid across and straightened up and held in place. Then step by careful step, changing bearers when required, monitoring and talking to Gary all the way, we convey our gift-wrapped patient along the tunnel to the bottom of the lift. The initial urgency of the scenario has settled into a methodical calm, and although the journey is slow and inelegant, it's a world away from the prospect of getting him up the spiral stairs. Only once we've laid the stretcher down at the other end does the site manager remember he has a small motorised cart that we could have used. We all try not to think too hard about this.

Up the lift, outside and onto the truck, which has been moved up the road, and Gary and his flail chest are whisked away to the trauma centre and a waiting team of experts for repair. I don't know where this leaves my pessimists, but with the right care Gary should be fine.

There's a curious moment of stillness when the ambulance is gone. Within minutes, the street has cleared. Exhilaration fades to silence. I walk back above ground to the original scene to collect my equipment: it's still down there some-where. Still in the pit, for all I know.

But someone's been a bit too efficient: the yard is deserted and the gates are locked. It's just gone three a.m. and my kit is sixty feet underground. I run my hand through my hair and it comes back thick with soot. Time to find someone with a key . . .

VI

There's nothing like a dose of recklessness for focusing the mind. Four months into my training and yet to be found out, as I can't help but think of it, on placement with a seasoned crew who are steering my first tentative steps, trusted to see patients but not yet charged with their care, I still can't shake the sensation of someone who's won a world cruise but forgotten to renew his passport.

22-YR-OLD MALE, HANGING

So far I've sampled the thrills of blue-light driving (that novelty won't last long) and attended a selection of reassuringly underwhelming calls. An anaphylactic reaction turns out to be tingly lips and a tight throat. An unconscious young woman has merely swooned. A child with breathing problems is a 'hot baby' – an infant with an untreated fever. Such jobs are happily within my comfort zone, and I start to feel that maybe I can do this after all. But I know I need to get my teeth into something a bit more catastrophic – while I'm still under someone's guidance and don't have to be in charge.

NEAR HANGING. CUT DOWN BY FATHER

It's night and the roads are surprisingly clear. There's a tendency for new recruits to race to everything, high on the velocity of heroism, but I try not to get carried away. I'm still getting used to the fluid nature of how jobs appear on our dispatch screen (or MDT): since the calls are often still incoming, things can change radically, even veering from a cardiac arrest to a cancellation, within seconds.

PATIENT BREATHING. FAMILY ON SCENE

It's hard to tell how unwell this patient will be: what's described on the screen is often a very different scenario from what we find when we arrive.

TRAUMA TEAM EN RTE, PLS REPORT ON ARRIVAL

We grab our initial equipment and cross the car park to the flats. A fast-response car pulls up; the police are close behind.

A man of about sixty ushers us towards a small bedroom. He's clutching a belt, and his eyes are wide and raw. I hear screaming from down the hall. Across the doorframe there's a chin-up bar you have to duck under to get in, and just inside the room, on the floor, lies a young man with a shaved head. His face and head are maroon – the colour your finger goes if you wind string around and hold it tight. He's breathing, but noisily, as if something coarse is scraping his insides.

The others move seamlessly into action. One feels for a pulse, holds the head, lifts the chin. The patient doesn't react. Another plugs in an oxygen mask and hands it to the first. The third guides the father into the hall, asks him calmly what happened. For a moment I just stand and stare, not frozen exactly, but not quite up to speed with my colleagues. They're moving so intuitively, as if they've worked this exact scenario many times before, and I'm still taking it all in and wondering what's actually occurred. In my head I'm thinking *Airway, Breathing, Circulation* – but the guys around me are several steps ahead.

Can you pass me a Guedel, mate?

I look at him blankly. I know what this is. I just need a moment.

An OP. An OP airway?

Of course. A Guedel. An OP.

Oh. Sure.

The little claw-shaped device that hooks the tongue away from the back of the throat and opens up the airway.

What colour?

Let's try a pink.

I rummage in the oxygen bag. Naturally, pink is the only colour I can't see.

Any joy?

Sorry. No pink.

Orange then.

Errr . . .

Just pass me the bag if you like.

But I find an orange and pass it across. He slides it into the patient's mouth and spins it round – the breathing quietens slightly.

Right. We need some obs. Can you pass me the defib?

I grab the machine and swing it across towards him, but

I'm a bit too eager in the heat of the moment, and it crashes into the frame of the bed with a clang.

Easy tiger! Let's keep it calm. No need to rush.

Sorry.

Let's have some sats and a blood pressure. Can you hook up the end-tidal?

Oxygen saturations and blood pressures I've been doing all week; the end-tidal I'm not so sure about. I've been shown it once, but never put it on an actual patient. It's a little bit of tubing that hooks under the nose, and measures the carbon dioxide coming out of the patient's lungs. I pull open the pockets of the machine, hoping I'll know it when I see it.

How we doing?

I can't see one here.

Check that top pocket.

I unzip it. Ah.

That's it, mate. Now plug it in and hook it up.

I try to unwind the tubing but it gets tangled instead, and suddenly I have a handful of knots. I push one end back through the jumble but that just makes it worse.

Sorry . . .

Then the hand of my mentor appears holding a second, disentangled specimen. I plug it in and try to hook it round the patient's nose and ears, but by now my fingers have got butterflies and of course it gets stuck and won't quite stretch to the second ear, so I tug it a bit tighter and pull off the first.

Take your time, buddy . . .

The responder reaches down and loosens the toggle and now it's long enough. Haste and speed. I secure it in place.

Our colleague has got some history from the patient's dad. Apparently the patient sent his friend some worrying text messages. The friend tried to call him back but no one was answering.

Fortunately she had his dad's number. She couldn't get through to start with. But when she did, he rushed in here and cut him down.

He used the belt?

On the bar.

Okay, let's update the trauma team. And we're gonna need some gear from the truck.

He turns to me.

Think you can manage?

Sure.

Okay. Suction, scoop, blocks, straps. Trolley if it'll fit through the doors.

I head to the door. My mentor catches my eye.

Want a hand?

I shake my head.

I'll be fine.

See if you can get the truck a bit closer.

Sure.

The trauma team are pulling up when I get outside.

Where we going, mate?

Errr . . .

I turn to point them through the doors – just as a police officer appears:

This way, gents. Follow me.

★

I never actually hit the floor on that fateful first day. I gulped down the nausea and fixed my eyes on a point in the distance, and eventually the brain-fog cleared and I made it to the end – physically unscathed, emotionally spent, but with a lingering sense that I didn't really belong here, that I had taken the seat of someone far more deserving.

Through my early training I maintained a low profile: studying hard, keeping my head down and trying to pre-empt anything that might set me off again. I practised chest compressions on dummies and tried to memorise Boyle's law; I learnt about different types of fracture and the situations in which the emergency medicines should, and should not, be administered. If not an outright phobia, I uncovered a mild distrust of blood outside the body (a little impractical, perhaps, but not without logic), and of course a rich terror of anything to do with childbirth, cultivated in the customary way during school sex-ed classes and brought spectacularly to bloom in the delivery suite encounter I've already described. But if I knew something along these lines was coming, I could steel myself and make sure I was well prepared, on the basis that being forewarned was to be forearmed, and hoping that gradual exposure and familiarity would lead to a newfound poise in relation to all things obstetric and/or haematological.

Apart from the day I was blindsided by the graphic explanation of how a dialysing fistula is created, which induced a pallid nausea that threatened to undo all my careful planning, my strategy seemed, on the whole, to succeed. Whether this would count for anything once I was out of the classroom and faced with real patients, real blood, real fistulae, remained to be seen.

Was I being foolhardy? Irresponsible? Would members of the public be horrified if they knew that their critically ill loved ones were soon to be left in the hands of someone who swooned at the first mention of haemoglobin? Perhaps. But I retained a pretty strong belief that humans are nothing if not adaptable, and that in the right conditions we have the ability to conquer our minor demons and master new skills that were previously beyond our reach. I'd seen plenty of episodes of *Faking It* that seemed to prove my point. I'd watched cricketers win *Strictly Come Dancing* and film stars become politicians. If the Terminator could end up as Governor of California, surely I could get over a few bodily terrors. This was, after all, why I'd joined the job: to see if I could grasp something apparently beyond my reach. So long as I didn't leave a trail of destruction and disaster in my wake . . .

Suction, scoop, blocks and straps. Suction, scoop, blocks and straps. Trolley if I can get it in. I repeat the mantra so I won't forget.

I gather the equipment and dump it on the bed: the collars and straps and the rigid metal stretcher we call a scoop. But I can't find the head blocks. I rifle through the cupboards – am I looking in the right place? Why does this sort of thing always happen to the novice? I've been told you can roll a blanket to emulate blocks – but I don't know how, and maybe that kind of improvisation is frowned upon around here.

I try to remove the suction from its mount, but the catch

is stiff and it won't come away. I've been shown the equipment in a classroom, but it wasn't attached to the wall of an ambulance then. Is there a secret knack? I try it from a different angle, pull the lever the other way, but it doesn't shift and then there's a loud cracking sound. Oh dear.

Time is ticking and I don't want to be the newbie who's sent on a routine errand and never returns. I turn my attention to moving the truck – which is easier said than done. Every man and his dog seems to have turned up to this incident, and the streets are swarming with blue-light vehicles, including a second ambulance which must have snuck up while I was wrestling with the suction. I swing the truck forward and turn the nose into a gap, then pull back round to reverse towards the entrance, but there's a pillar in the way. I give it two more attempts, heaving the wheel clockwise, anti-clockwise, before I realise it's not going to happen; there's just not enough room – and now I'm pretty much stuck. That scene from *Austin Powers* flashes through my mind and I decide to cut my losses and pull back out – which is easier said than done after working so hard to get into the gap in the first place. It takes me several minutes, and all I've achieved at the end of my struggles is a return to my starting point.

I lower the back, pull out the bed and give the suction one more go. It comes away from the wall as easily as you like – what was all the fuss about? I drag and push the trolley bed towards the entrance, stretching forward to stop the precious cargo from tumbling off the edge of the path, and skirting round the sides to keep it from careening onto the grass. Eventually I get it to the doors and apply the brakes. How long have I been gone? Hopefully they've been busy with the patient and won't even have noticed.

I load myself up with the gear and head inside. But I don't get very far, because I'm met by a dozen uniformed emergency workers coming the other way: ambulance, police and trauma team, bearing aloft the patient, collared, strapped, blocked and blanketed in apparatus from ambulance number two. I throw myself against the wall just to get out of the way. While all the inspiration and heroism has been occurring inside, I've been busy manoeuvring an ugly yellow box around in the dark.

At the back of the convoy are my mentor and his crewmate.

Ah! The wanderer returns!

Have a nice trip?

We'd forgotten what you looked like.

Not got bored and gone home?

I would come to learn that ambulance crews like to keep things simple: free from grey areas, unburdened by doubt. Temperamentally drawn to clarity and action, we tend to go straight for the jugular, reducing complex scenarios to instinctive decisions for a rapid response. A delay to consider the nuances or weigh up the light and the shade might have serious consequences, so the tendency is always to treat for the worst and consider the niceties at a later date.

This kind of response demands a certain amount of self-possession: you have to step into an unknown situation and take control, be willing to make your mistakes in public, and not be afraid to tread on a few toes. In the heat of the moment, there's little time for hand-wringing and introspection – or making your parking look neat.

One of my tutors suggested I'd struggle with this part of the job, having spotted a diffident nature and a tendency to caution when action was required. He was right. Part of this was prudence – I was already fearful of being caught out. But part of it lay deeper, innately, and while I was convinced I could get better at the mechanics of emergency care, something in me resisted the prospect of doing so while trying to forge a more forceful, authoritative facsimile of myself. Was it possible to find another approach?

VII

Reggie's on the floor and he can't get up. He's in the bathroom, wedged between the toilet and his wheelchair. It was light when he fell, but that was two hours ago and now he's lying in the dark. He's held on as long as he could, but now his jogging bottoms are soaked through and his skin is starting to burn. He's tried to haul himself up using the bowl and the rails fitted to his bathroom walls, but his arms are shrivelled to frailty these days. At least he was wearing his pendant and could reach the button to raise the alarm.

Reggie's waiting for someone to lift him out of the mire. In the prime of his life, he's as helpless as a child. He's forty-six years old.

Ninety minutes ago we were on our way. Then we got cancelled and sent to a twenty-one-year-old who was 'unconscious and struggling to breathe'. When we arrived she was lying on the floor with her eyes closed. She'd had an argument with her boyfriend. Her family were terrified because she wouldn't answer their questions, wouldn't move, wouldn't react. So they called 999.

After we've spent an hour on scene, coaching her breathing, ruling out the red flags, interceding with the family, harmony seems to be restored. And when we make ourselves available again, Reggie's address reappears on our screen.

We retrieve the key from the keysafe outside and call out as we enter. We follow Reggie's voice to the bathroom and switch on the light. The extractor fan starts to whir.

You took your sweet time.

I'm really sorry.

Is it your fault?

Well . . . We got sent somewhere else.

Don't apologise then.

Okay. But I'm sorry you've been waiting so long. How long ago did you fall?

I don't even know. What does it matter? Here I am.

Reggie's been superseded. Abandoned by a system skewed to overstatement. Yet he delivers these words, not as a simmering rebuke from the cold, forgotten night, but in a flat monotone, with a weariness that suggests he's been a low-priority emergency call before. It's like he's reading out someone else's lines; as if he lacks the energy to get mad.

Okay. Let's get you up.

Before we move Reggie, we ask how he fell, whether he banged his head, if he was knocked out or has pain in his neck – all the greatest hits of patient assessment – but Reggie's impatient to skip to the end.

Forget all that. Just get me off the floor.

We move the wheelchair out and slide Reggie into the middle of the room. It's a square box modified for his

predicament, with grip bars and concertina panels and a futuristic wipe-clean floor. He's gone rigid in the shape of a
question mark, his stringy muscles in spasm, like a giant
embryo with a wispy beard. We lift him into a sitting position; he's as light as a cardboard cut-out of himself. His vest
hangs off his shoulders like a dress; his jogging bottoms billow
around his stick legs; you could hang a rack of shirts from
his clavicles. This is what people mean when they describe
someone as a shadow of their former self: Reggie's body is
unadorned information, a news report of its previous shape,
factually sound but devoid of local colour. A physique of
nouns but no adjectives.

We peel away Reggie's clothes. His limbs move routinely
into position to allow it.

Do you have carers, Reggie?

Reggie nods.

How often do they come?

Twice a day.

Morning and evening?

Reggie nods.

What are they like?

He shrugs. They're carers. What do we want him to say?

Do you get out much?

Not recently.

No?

He takes a deep breath.

It's a lot of effort.

Of course.

I'd rather stay in.

71

The skin on Reggie's elbows and hips is cherry-red from rubbing against the vinyl flooring. His flesh is pimpled in the cold, the hairs standing on end. His thighs are damp with urine and his buttocks are smeared with excrement. These are simple matters of fact; no comment is made.

We find some wipes and clean the worst of the mess away. My crewmate turns on the shower and holds his gloved hand under the water until it runs hot. We lift Reggie off the floor and place him on the shower seat, redirect the spray so that the water falls on his shoulders and cascades down his skeletal torso. His body starts to relax and after a couple of minutes he can hold onto one of the bars and support himself.

What about family, Reggie?

What about them?

Do you have any?

I do.

Are they near by?

I grew up round here. All my family are near by.

You see them much?

No.

They don't come round?

He shakes his head.

You want us to call anyone?

Why?

Tell them what's happened?

He shakes his head.

We lift Reggie from the seat into a kind of standing pose. He's leaning forward, with his arms hooked around my neck like we're about to dance, while I hold him at the waist, which means my hands are practically inside his ribcage. It looks like an embrace between two men worried their bodies might accidentally touch. Which, sort of, it is.

My crewmate takes the shower head off the wall and trains the jet of water onto Reggie's xylophone back, then down to his hollowed out buttocks, between his legs, his elongated thighs. The force of the water is relentless, invasive, purging. He soaks a flannel and adds shower gel and begins daubing Reggie's skin methodically from high to low.

Reggie holds on, unspeaking. Is he thinking of a very different time in his life? He has shelves of vinyl and decks in the next room: did Reggie DJ to crowds of people in his past life? In the corner of the lounge a rowing machine is folded upright and gathering dust; draped with coats and jumpers that surely no longer fit him: how long can it be since Reggie did any kind of workout?

The flannel comes away dark, humiliated. It's washed clean under the water and relathered, and the scrubbing resumes. Again it's discoloured, washed, reapplied. Now we rinse: foam and excrement and grime cascade down to the floor and are chased to the plughole in the corner by the stream of water. We lower Reggie onto the shower seat again and let the water run over him until the steam fills the room and clouds the mirror, and the smells of lime and mint saturate the air with the promise of cleanliness.

One of us scouts around the flat and finds an enormous towel shedding fluff, along with some boxers, a faded Bob Marley T-shirt and some checked pyjama bottoms. We drape the towel round Reggie's shoulders and fold it in front of his body and he's engulfed. Of course it looks like a shroud, but it also gives him an air of tranquillity. With the pitiless truth of his body hidden away, his face looks more nourished, more animated. His cheeks have some colour from the heat of the shower; his eyes have let in some light.

Better?

He nods. There are tiny strands of towel-fuzz caught on his beard and the straggly hairs around his throat.

Thank you.

It's nothing. Seriously.

Well. Yeah.

Reggie, do you want a cup of tea?

He shakes his head.

Coffee?

Nah, man.

Something to eat?

I don't eat too much, you know.

Understood. Shall we help you get dressed?

Give me a minute.

Of course.

We give Reggie a minute. Drops of water fall from the shower head to the floor. PLIP . . . PLIP . . . PLIP . . .

I see my sister, you know.

Yeah?

She comes to see me. (PLIP.) *She's the only one.* (PLIP.) *I don't blame them. I wouldn't visit. I burned a lot of bridges. Ha! Would you believe I used to be tough?*

He shivers – it's practically a shudder, and he almost falls off the seat.

A real tough guy. Huh!

You sure you don't want us to call her?

Nahhh. Just get me dressed. And I ain't goin' to no hospital.

We help him stand again, hold him straight. I dry his legs and privates.

Where d'you wanna go now, Reggie?

The chair in there.

The recliner?

He nods. We wrap the towel around his waist and sit him on the shower seat. He scoops his hands around his thigh and hauls his lifeless left foot off the ground. I bend down and hook the boxers onto the ankle. Reggie lifts his right leg in the same way and I hook the boxers again. I scrunch the pyjamas up into a figure of eight and we repeat the process, though it's more effort this time. Then we stand Reggie up and drag the elastic waist bands of his boxers and trousers up to his hips. But when we let go, the garments drop straight to his ankles and land in two hoops in a puddle on the floor.

Oh! Sorry. Sorry.

I drop down to Reggie's feet and grab the clothes and try to hoist them back up, but there's an absence of flesh for the elastic to cling onto. Somehow this feels like a bigger indignity than before, as if we've played a playground prank on him. I slide the trousers up, take a fistful of material at Reggie's midriff and hold it in place to keep them from dropping again.

I'm really sorry. We'll get you some dry ones.

Forget it.

No, really, they're all wet.

They're fine. It happens every time.

You're sure?

There's safety pins on the side there. The carers leave them. It happens every time.

Sure enough, beside the sink I find a pair of oversized safety pins. While my crewmate keeps Reggie vertical, I gather a large flap of pyjama cloth and fold it back over itself and secure the pin to fashion Reggie a pair of what they used to call hoisties. This gives the trousers the look of an umbrella that's opened halfway and then changed its mind: the cuffs dangle above the ankles, while at the hips they mushroom outwards and then dive back in to a narrow loop at belly-button height. They're a canvas sack in search of a gastric band, a morbid reminder of how far Reggie's illness has cut him off from the outside world.

I can picture Reggie as a snappy dresser. Maybe a bit of a ladies' man. Perhaps he got in a bit of trouble from time to time, drank in the bars round the corner, or played at some of the local clubs. Now he's reduced to being dressed by two strangers in hand-me-downs from his former self, a big brother he'll never catch up with because he's shrinking not growing, held together with safety pins and unable to wash himself clean.

This is surely the final insult for anyone like Reggie: the moment vanity dies. Any sense of taking pride in one's physical appearance is sacrificed to the all-conquering will of practicality, where fashions and preferences get no look-in, and the physical form that was once an outward narrative of what's inside becomes a simple host for biological processes.

No longer is the body an emblem of vitality or discipline, even of gluttony or indolence; no longer is it a signifier of sex or strength or style; of success or shame. Now it's simply a thing that falls and needs to be lifted, gets hungry and needs to be fed; an apparatus that gets cold and needs to be heated, that gets dirty and needs to be cleaned – in the most convenient way possible.

The best we can do is drape Bob Marley and his giant spliff over Reggie's coat-hanger shoulders, before we help him back into his chair and wheel him into the lounge.

What time is it?

Quarter past eleven.

You know what? Just take me to my bed. I'm done.

So we wheel Reggie to his bed and help him stand and turn and sit and lie down on his side. We put his pendant back round his neck and pull the covers over him and turn off the light.

We've given Reggie no emergency treatment. We've solved no medical mysteries. We've averted no disasters. But this is the most useful I've felt in a long time.

Thanks, gents. You've been princes.

It's nothing.

Listen, on the way out?

Yep?

Can you switch on that radio?

Of course.

VIII

No one wants a reputation as a sucker. This is a point of pride in most professions, but in the fertile soil of emergency care it's practically a mantra. Even a couple of months into my new identity, I've learnt that much.

Don't ever let them take the piss. You show a sign of weakness and they'll have you for breakfast.

I was given this advice on my first placement. At first I wasn't sure who it referred to – the patients, the radio dispatcher, the other drivers on the road? Maybe humanity in general? My mentor seemed to have a beef with most of these groups, so it was hard to narrow down, and I was too intimidated to ask.

However, I was determined to give people the benefit of the doubt. At least until I had a reason to think otherwise. I wasn't totally naïve. I knew there'd be difficult individuals and situations that were not what they appeared. I'd seen those episodes of *House* in which heartless Hugh Laurie sneers that all patients are liars – and is spectacularly vindicated in the final act. I'd been told all the stories – about patients playing the system, out to waste your time, offloading their elderly relatives, trying to jump the queue at A&E, looking to make trouble, trying to get their fix. I'd listened to the mess-room cynics luxuriating in their hard-earned misanthropy. I'd met plenty of chancers already, and delivered them timidly to thin-lipped triage nurses who'd seen it all before and didn't even look up from what they were doing, too tired to hide their contempt for either the patient or their escort in green.

Yet I was adamant none of this would get me down. People just needed to be given a chance, I felt sure. A fair hearing and a bit of attention. It was all about attitude, surely. I didn't want to be gullible, but neither did I want to assume the worst. I felt confident that whatever occurred I could stick to my conviction that people are fundamentally good, and only difficult when things aren't going their way. Surely.

Our patient is sitting on a low wall next to an off-licence in the morning drizzle. Hood up, head down, tresses of wet hair scrawled across her face. As we pull up she spits into a puddle, then clutches her stomach and doubles over in pain. There's something familiar about that movement.

A man on a mobile phone is sitting beside her, but he stands and walks off down the road at our approach. She shouts something at his back. Without turning he throws down his arm as if he's flicking something from his hand.

We get out of the truck. My crewmate kicks off with a cheerful melody:

Hi there! Shall we get straight on?
I can't get up.

Just a few steps? We'll help you.

I need some gas.

The patient's eyes are closed, her face an elaborate frown.

What gas?

Gas and air.

You've had it before?

She nods.

Let's get you out of the rain and sorted out.

She opens her eyes:

I'm already wet. Who you worried about, yourself or me?

Don't you want to get in the warm?

She looks straight at my crewmate and spits on the floor.

I'm not moving without the gas.

We exchange a look. I fetch the gas.

Is this even on? I don't think it's working.

She holds up the mouthpiece.

It's definitely working.

Can you check it?

She's sucking great gulps of gas into her lungs.

It's working, trust me.

Today her name's Annabel, but I've met her before, a couple of weeks ago, and then her name was Selina. She's wearing running trainers without socks, baggy jogging bottoms and an enormous hoodie, as if she's just been to the gym but come home in someone else's clothes. Her hands are grubby and her eyes are fringed with yesterday's mascara. My mind flits back to that gentleman walking off as we arrived, and I wonder who he was and where he's disappeared to.

Well it's not helping. I don't feel any different.

Tell us what's happened, Annabel. Point to where it hurts.

I can sense my crewmate's good humour being put to the test. She does the talking while I attach the machinery. Annabel knows the routine: she puts out her finger for the probe that reads her oxygen levels and her pulse, and pulls up her sleeve for the BP cuff:

It's like someone's stabbing me. Burning me. Squeezing my ribs. This gas isn't working. I think I need something stronger.

Up her arm I see the same tiny bruises and scabs as before. They follow the line of her veins. I wrap the cuff round her skinny arm and it inflates. She sucks on the gas again.

When did it start? Have you had it before?

Loads of times.

Really?

But never as bad as this.

Have you taken anything?

She shakes her head:

All my tablets are at home.

Where's that?

Does it matter?

What d'you normally take?

None of it works.

It's a sparring match: my crewmate pushing for specifics; Annabel falling back on the visible testimony of her suffering. But my crewmate's persistent – not mean, but determined:

So it's an ongoing problem? What's the diagnosis?

Babe, it's really hurting. Why all the questions?

I'm sorry, Annabel. Have they told you what the problem is?

You know I'm in pain, don't you? What else do you need to know?

Do you have a letter from the hospital maybe?

Do I look like I've got a letter from the hospital?

We need to know where the pain's coming from. Will you let me examine your abdomen?

I'm telling you it's serious, babe, what more do you need?

We want to give you the most appropriate treatment.

Annabel stares hard at my crewmate. Is it possible she's being too harsh? Would I be more tolerant if I was the one doing the talking? Or more pliable perhaps? It's clear to both of us that Annabel's having a bad time of it – maybe not a medical emergency, but an ongoing struggle. All we'll ever get in these encounters is a glimpse, a snapshot, but the signs are there, and I still have that urge to give her the benefit of the doubt.

My sense of generosity takes a blow when Annabel, with a rapid sweep of the arm, throws the mouthpiece on the floor; then she begins retching, writhing in her seat and growling throatily:

Heeugghhh! Heeee-ughhhh!

I open the cupboard and hold out a cardboard vomit bowl.

Here you go.

She clutches at her belly with one hand and then, with the other, pushes all four fingers into her mouth and as far down her throat as she can. Her eyes widen as her body convulses in a red-faced spasm. She heaves herself forward, then back, then forward again. I hold out the bowl under her face and put my hand on her shoulder.

Try not to force it, Annabel.

She slams the vomit bowl away from her, crushing it against my chest, then leans to the side, pauses, and expectorates a massive globule of yellow bile and saliva onto the ambulance floor.

Haaaaarrrrggghhhh!!

She shudders involuntarily.

Are you okay?

A thin stalactite of spittle dangles from her bottom lip to the floor. She swats it away and wipes her hand on the edge of the chair, then leans back in the seat, exhausted. I hand her a tissue. She wipes her face, then drops the tissue on the floor beside the gobbet of sputum. She looks at us each in turn.

Sorry about your ambulance.

Last time I came to Annabel/Selina, she was in her flat, surrounded by boxes of meds she said weren't touching the pain. Pancreatitis, she said. My crewmate that day gave her IV morphine and anti-sickness and we took her in, but when we got to A&E the nurse sighed like she'd been punctured with a giant pin. Selina had been there every day that week, and each time had left after she'd been given all the medication she was going to get, but before they'd had a chance to complete the assessment, only to turn up again the next day. Recently she'd started getting aggressive when she was told there was no morphine coming her way.

She's given no indication that she recognises me from before, but I doubt she'd say if she did. If she's after something similar today, she still has a few tricks up her sleeve:

You're a paramedic, right?

She's looking at my crewmate's shoulder.

That's right.

So you've got morphine . . .

You've had morphine before?

You wouldn't want to deny me treatment, would you?

Sorry?

Don't you have, like, a duty of care?

How do you mean?

If I tell you I need morphine, you have to give it to me.

No. I need to use my clinical judgement. Morphine's a serious medicine.

You're not a doctor.

No.

So none of that shit matters. I'm in pain and I'm telling you I need morphine.

It would be irresponsible of me to give morphine to someone just because they asked for it.

But I'm in pain. You can see I'm in pain.

Okay. The hospital's less than a mile away. We'll be there in five minutes.

No no no! You can't take me there.

Why not?

Not there. You gotta take me somewhere else.

What's wrong with the local hospital?

They don't treat me right. They're shitty. They palm me off.

When were you last there?

Listen, babe, that doesn't matter. You can't feel my pain, can you?

When were you last at the hospital?

I'm in a shitload of pain and you're denying me pain relief.

Let's get you moving.

You're not listening to me, babe. I'm telling you I'm in pain.

You can have some gas on the way.

Have you ever heard the saying that the pain belongs to the patient, not the paramedic? Didn't they teach you that in training school?

I'm sorry?

I said, 'The pain belongs to the patient, not the paramedic.'

Where's she heard this from? A doctor? Another paramedic? Has she read it in a medical textbook?

You can't tell me how much pain I'm in.

Okay. Let's go.

So I think you better take my word for it and give me some morphine. I think that's your job.

Paramedics don't tend to make great claims about their clinical expertise, but there are certain skills they consider their forte. One of these is recognising a really sick patient at first glance. Another is detecting the scent of a charlatan from about three streets away.

I've heard colleagues joke guiltily about how cynical they've become; how they've grown to doubt what they're told or distrust some patients' motives; how they pay more attention to the involuntary clues than the story they're told; how they can anticipate the course of most jobs before they even arrive on scene.

The dangers of doubting people's motives in the clinical setting are obvious. If you can't trust the patient, who can you rely on for your information? Any kind of prejudgement can send you down the wrong path – and it's dangerous and embarrassing if you have to retreat and try a different track.

But cynicism breaks both ways, and there's something more sinister at play in this scenario: the type of cynicism that uses the misfortune of others for its own advantage. It's a behaviour that seems to flourish in the ambiguous one-off encounters of ambulance care.

An example? When a patient says they want to go to hospital by ambulance so they won't have to wait so long at A&E, they're being cynical without even knowing it. Ambulance crews and call-takers hear this repeatedly; that patients want to go in by ambulance because they'll be seen more quickly. It's a myth – ambulance patients are fed into the same triage stream as everyone else; treatment depends on clinical need not mode of arrival – but this doesn't stop people trying their luck. Most people would agree that emergency ambulances should be available for critically ill patients, not to facilitate queue-jumping; so why do so many seemingly reasonable and informed people make this request without blinking an eye?

In any walk of life, someone who has to accommodate the manipulative behaviours of others is liable to start anticipating those behaviours as a result: it's not a matter of being pessimistic or mean-spirited, it's simple pragmatism. When you're dealing with something of a loose cannon, it can be wise to put on some protective armour.

So, we've brought Annabel to the local hospital, and she's not happy, not happy at all. When I open the back door, she stays stubbornly in the seat, soggy shoes up on the trolley bed. She shows no sign now of being in pain.

Come on, Annabel, let's go and see the nurse.

No.

We can't stay here all day, can we?

Take me somewhere else then.

That's not going to happen.

It's at this point that Annabel stands up in the middle of the ambulance, slides her trousers down to her ankles, squats unsteadily – and urinates profusely onto the ambulance floor.

You couldn't say the warning signs weren't there. Once it was clear she wasn't getting her way, Annabel's objections became nastier, her movements more threatening. When she finally stood from the chair, I sensed her anger was about to turn destructive. The relocation of the trousers stopped me in my tracks for a moment – but that purposeful crouch, like a squat in the woods, was a call to arms.

In an instant, all my good intentions go up in smoke. I see what Annabel is about to do. I remember the ambulance is on a forward slope, and anticipate the direction of the impending stream.

Our bags! Our bags! Get them off the floor!

It's a badge of honour for ambulance crews never to appear panicked or rushed, but there are a few exceptions, and one of them is when your packed lunch is about to be over-whelmed by a torrent of your patient's wee. My crewmate hoists our bags up just as the steaming flood approaches. The sour perfume of fermented fruit fills the air. I grab a stack of incontinence pads and throw them, past the patient, for my crewmate to scatter liberally over the sodden floor before the contaminating flow reaches the cab. She distributes them in a hasty semi-circle like a croupier, then nudges them with her foot into a kind of absorbent dam, making sure nothing will pass.

Annabel is still peeing. Either she's consumed a substantial liquid breakfast or she has a bladder of steel. When her liquid protest is over she repositions her trousers and retakes her seat. She refuses to leave the ambulance unless we take her to a different hospital.

We're stuck.

We inform Control of the situation. They don't quite understand. They have a screen full of calls to fulfil, and can't comprehend why a crew who are already at hospital can't just get their patient inside.

We ask the hospital security for assistance – and you can guess how keen they are to help us bring a urine-drenched troublemaker into their overloaded department. We might be sitting outside a working A&E, but our encounter with Annabel is far from over. My good intentions are battered and bruised. I can just see Hugh Laurie's sardonic frown.

No doubt it would have been easier to give Annabel what she wanted. Perhaps it would have been the right thing to do – though I don't think so. In the moments when negative expectations are played out so flawlessly, it's as if one brand of cynicism has nurtured another. Either way, it turns out that, when you're trying to remove your personal belongings from the vengeful tide of a patient's urine, expecting the worst can sometimes have its uses.

IX

We're delayed getting to Samuel because of the traffic. The traffic's stacked because the road is closed. And the road's closed because Samuel's lying in the middle of the junction, flat on his back, with a police officer pushing rhythmically on his chest.

When we pull up, the first responder's already on scene. His car and three police vehicles are distributed around the junction, boots open, lights flickering. There's a small crowd holding up camera phones. It's not their relative lying in the road, so it's a fascinating little mystery for them, a prime-time drama on their doorstep, a story to tell. The police are keeping them back on the pavement – which makes it all the more exciting.

Samuel's car sits sideways across the lane, its bonnet crumpled inwards as if it's been punched in the belly. One of the traffic lights leans awkwardly askew and a bollard has been knocked across the road. There's a wide stretch of cross-hatched tarmac, and Samuel's body straddles three yellow squares.

A matter of minutes ago, Samuel collided with the traffic island in front of a police car parked on the corner. When the officers approached they found he wasn't breathing, so they pulled him out and started CPR right there in the road. It might not look it now, but today Samuel is just about the luckiest man on the planet.

He's in his fifties, and solidly built. His shirt's been cut off, the defibrillator's beside him and the pads are going on as we approach. There's no immediate sign of an injury. The oxygen is set up with the bag-valve mask, and the officers are counting their compressions and stopping at thirty so the first responder can give two breaths.

At the next break everyone peers at the defib screen. The line is jagged, disordered, erratic: this patient's heart is in a rhythm called ventricular fibrillation (VF). It's weak – or 'fine' – but shockable. This is good news. The first responder pushes charge and adds a few more compressions and everyone steps back.

Everyone stand clear! Oxygen away!

He hits the button and the shock is delivered. It's less of a boom and more of a jolt: the patient's body pops and settles in a rapid single convulsion, as if someone's poked him with a sharp stick when he was drifting off to sleep. But there's no break in the process:

Back on the chest, please, guys. Can someone else take a turn?

Sure. No problem.

A second officer moves into position; the compressions recommence.

Samuel's heart has stopped doing its job, so the rest of his body is shutting down. It has one simple task: to contract, about once a second, every second, for the rest of Samuel's life. But it's not contracting; it's quivering. So, for now, the police officer's arms are Samuel's external heart.

This quivering is the result of the arrhythmia, the VF. Commonly caused by death of heart tissue, such as occurs in a heart attack, ventricular fibrillation is the dissident cousin of that familiar ECG trace you'll have seen on a hundred medical textbooks and TV credit sequences. Instead of a repetitive cycle of depolarising bumps and spikes, it creates a chaotic sequence of futile electrical signals, a landscape of foothills but no mountains, so that the heart trembles like a jelly when it should squeeze. The result is an absence of circulation.

Every two minutes we check the rhythm. The shape of the lines on the screen tells us if the electrical activity is viable – organised to stimulate a spontaneous contraction, capable of creating a pulse, compatible with life – and, if not, if the rhythm requires defibrillation. Twice more we stop CPR to check, and twice more out on the tarmac Samuel's heart is pummelled with a shock.

We insert a cannula in his vein; we place airway adjuncts into his mouth and nose. We fetch more oxygen and a trolley and a blanket and a lifting stretcher. Meanwhile the police officer keeps pushing on his chest:

One, two, three, four

Five, six, seven, eight –

like a metronome, until he reaches

– twenty-eight, twenty-nine, thirty –

and rests for a moment; the first responder lifts the patient's face into the mask and squeezes two breaths into his lungs; and the officer starts again.

We get a quick history of the crash: low-speed impact, minor damage, no one else involved; patient slumped at the wheel, no sign of an injury. In other words, it looks like the patient's had a collapse while driving which has caused the crash – and not the other way round. The implications start whirring: a sudden event, possibly cardiac in nature, no obvious precursors; a short down-time, a middle-aged patient, a quick response. All this points to a decent prognosis if we can break the cycle of VF and get the heart to beat of its own accord.

No one knows anything about the patient: where he lives, his age, his medical history, if he has any family; where he was going, and whether someone's waiting for him to arrive. Only later do we find out his name. He's overweight so he probably has high blood pressure, high cholesterol, possibly diabetes. High risk for a cardiac event. Was he driving himself to the doctor's, the hospital? Has he been unwell for days? Or did this event come out of the blue?

It's a warm, muggy day and beads of sweat are forming on the officer's forehead. They'll start dripping onto the patient soon. He'll be tired by now. The plan is to swap someone new onto the chest at the next rhythm check. But the switch never happens, because things are about to change.

There are good days and there are bad days – and there are days when you fall off a cliff. But then there are days when, by some tiny miracle of circumstance, exactly the right person just happens to be at the foot of that cliff, looking up with their arms outstretched. This is the kind of day Samuel is having.

Something very, very bad has happened to Samuel. We don't know it yet, but Samuel's had a myocardial infarction, a heart attack, severe enough to derange the electrics in his heart and stop it from beating. With no heartbeat there's no pulse, and with no pulse there's no circulation, and no oxygenation, and no breathing, and pretty soon no way out of the crematorium. Samuel has experienced a 'fatal' event.

Yet Samuel is not dead.

If Samuel's heart had stopped twelve hours earlier, his wife would likely have woken up next to a corpse. If he'd collapsed at home alone, he'd still be there now, quietly shuffling off this mortal coil. If he'd been driving down a country lane he might have put his car in a ditch and been discovered later, beyond help. On a motorway he might have caused a ten-car pile-up. There are any number of arbitrary variations which would transform Samuel's current plight. But Samuel suffered an attention-grabbing collapse in a very public place, right in front of someone who had the skills to intervene, within minutes of his catastrophic event. And that, for Samuel, is about to make all the difference in the world.

This, right here, is the buzz. This is what I've been waiting for. Not the shootings and stabbings, not the pile-ups and one-unders and falls from heights. This is the moment. A patient whose outcome can be pulled from the flames. A future we might, in a single instant, transform. Not through inspiration or brilliance or ingenuity, but by following a simple algorithm honed on the successes and failures of the past; not on our own, but as part of a chain of advocates working towards one goal.

Is it wrong to be exhilarated? To feel a kind of excitement? Shocking a heart from a fatal arrhythmia back to a working rhythm is the simplest thing we do. It takes just a few seconds. It requires little skill. That's what all those defibrillators in local shopping centres and train stations are all about. Yet in certain circumstances (and, I have to stress, not all cases), it can make the biggest difference it's possible to make.

My early months on the road have been a contraflow of instruction and disposal. I've undergone a rapid education in how the theory of this job interacts with its reality, a place where the clinical portion seems to shrink, or even become completely obscured – and at the same time, through exposure to a complex variety of workaday crises, I've found some of my original learning slipping out of my mind. It's as if, for every anxiety attack I've coached to tranquillity, and every parent I've introduced to Calpol, I've let go of one of the underlying physical laws or pharmacological reactions I worked so hard, just a few months ago, to understand so I could pass my exams.

I've grown used to making marginal impacts. I've discovered that many of the situations I'm expected to intervene in are neither critical nor even medical in nature. Sometimes I marvel at how a call has found its way to us. Sometimes I think I've forgotten my purpose.

And then I'm sent to someone like Samuel, and I remember why we're here.

At the third shock Samuel's future is turned upside down. Or, rather, one of many possible futures crash-lands into the present reality. In an instant the chaotic landscape of Samuel's heart trace, a jumble of fitful peaks and troughs, becomes an orderly cycle of bump–spike–hump–horizon, bump–spike–hump–horizon. It's like the background of an old cartoon on a loop, reassuringly repetitive – and just about the correct sequence to make the muscles contract.

We feel for a pulse and find one – at the throat and at the wrist. This is the Eureka moment. Samuel's heart is beating for itself.

Okay, we have a heartbeat, we have a nice strong pulse. Take a breather, mate. Let's do some obs and an ECG.

The officer sits back on his haunches and suddenly realises how warm it is. Someone passes him a bottle of water. He receives several pats on the back.

Well done, mate. Good work.

We connect the blood-pressure cuff, the pulse-ox, the ECG leads. The first paramedic keeps ventilating the lungs, all the while looking out for a spontaneous breath or other signs of life. He's tried to insert an advanced airway, but the patient won't tolerate having a large piece of plastic wedged into the back of his throat – another good sign.

The first trace we print out is still quite erratic – but clear enough to show a significant cardiac injury. It seems one of the arteries at the front of the heart has become blocked, killing some of the surrounding tissue, and causing the electrical disturbance that led to Samuel's collapse and crash. We will print off some clearer examples, but once we've stabilised the patient, we'll be taking him to the heart attack centre. They'll inject his coronary arteries with dye, clear any blockages and insert some tiny pieces of scaffolding to keep the pipes open and the muscle perfused. It could all be over in a couple of hours.

We load Samuel onto the ambulance and inform the hospital we're bringing him in. Things are looking better: he's even starting to breathe for himself. In the back with him are two medics and a constable.

But then, just as we pull away, Samuel's body twitches and the heart rhythm reverts to VF. A quick pulse check: he's back in cardiac arrest.

We pull over again – right beside Samuel's crashed car. This time he's already hooked up. The key here is an early shock: the quicker the intervention, the better the chance of reversion to a workable rhythm. There's no need for CPR: we confirm the rhythm and charge the pads. I reach out my finger to the big red button with the lightning strike logo.

Stand clear!

It's at this exact moment – just before I deliver the shock – that Samuel's body performs a sudden involuntary spasm, hinged at his waist, so that when the shock is delivered he's practically sitting up on the bed. Luckily he stops short of grabbing my arm. The force of the shock throws him back down; it also reverts his heart's electrics to an effective sinus rhythm: now his pulse is back and he's breathing again.

It's all over in seconds. After a pause to reassess, we set off again.

We proceed serenely for a time: no further arrhythmias pop up; no need for any more shocks. Then the patient's breathing becomes laboured, heavy, and he starts to shift irritably on the bed. Short involuntary bursts of tension seize his body, and squalid groans escape from his throat.

Samuel's mind is waking up from the strangest sleep it's ever experienced, and thick clouds of confusion are smothering his brain. Like a bear fighting a tranquilliser, he's bewildered, indignant, endlessly climbing a stairwell out of the basement of oblivion, never quite reaching ground-level. He lashes out at the daylight, but something holds him back. Voices harangue him in a language he can't decipher; his muscles strain to clear the horizon with brute force but they're outside his control; he kicks out at the darkness and his foot gets caught in something he can't identify. He's put it out of the window.

We update the hospital that the patient's become combative; he'll need sedation before any procedures can begin. We haul his leg in from the window before he loses his foot. The traffic is heavy in the afternoon heat. We keep him as still as we can for the remainder of the journey – mainly stopping him from hurting himself or us. We try to give him oxygen for his panicked brain, but he won't even accept the mask.

At the hospital we explain again about his agitation, but the staff don't seem too concerned. It's as if they don't quite believe us. We slide him onto the bed for the procedure and everyone but me steps away: I'm left gripping his hands at his waist. Suddenly free, Samuel's brain makes one final lurch for freedom, and he throws himself towards me and onto the floor.

Having seen for themselves, the staff call for an anaesthetist and the patient is sedated. They insert a wire into his wrist and feed it up to his heart and clear the blockage and reinflate the artery. They've performed this extraordinary, transformative procedure so often they could be darning socks.

In a few days, Samuel will be released from hospital. He'll embark on a part of his life he might never have reached. Will he feel like a lottery winner? A man reborn? A cheater of death? Will he feel a sense of responsibility? Or fear of what could or should have been?

As an ambulance crew we will never find out: we're on to our next patient within an hour and will never see Samuel again.

X

The man in the baseball cap and waistcoat is staring at the stack of newspapers. It comes up to his belly and is one of twelve equal piles. He removes his cap and rubs the top of his head with the heel of his hand.

You're sure it's necessary?

A hundred per cent.

His face is shielded by a thick bushy moustache and even thicker glasses perched on the end of his nose. His shirt stretches tight over his paunch, the tails untucked.

There must be another way.

I'm afraid not, sir.

He sighs profoundly, dramatically.

Fine.

With great care, he pinches the sides of the very top newspaper and lifts it from the pile. He delicately slides his hands underneath to hold it flat, as if he's dealing with an artefact that will crumble with any sudden movements. Then he stops. He's frozen for a moment. We wait.

Everything okay, sir?

He looks up at me, then at my colleague, then at his father, Patrick, through the doorway, inert on the bed. Then he looks back to the paper in his hands. What is he going to do with it? Take it into the other room? Return it to the top of the pile? Read the outdated front page? His breathing is quiet, his muscles tense. He seems to be agonising over the decision.

GnnnnhhhhNNNNHHHHH!

The sound starts as an irritated nasal whimper, and then sinks into a throaty roar: the pained groan of a brain in denial. Muscles that for all their effort can't find a solution.

What's happening, sir?

No response.

Sir?

Explain it to me again.

We need to get your dad downstairs. He can't walk so we're going to put him in a chair. But there's not enough room to get our chair along this passageway. I'm afraid we need you to move all these papers. Sir?

Right.

He seems distracted.

Do you understand what I'm saying?

Of course, of course. I'm not a fool. Of course I understand.

Good.

What about . . .? Can't you lift him?

Lift him how?

Over the newspapers?

In the chair?

Exactly.

In mid-air?

Well . . . Like this.

He demonstrates what he means with an imaginary load.

That wouldn't be safe. That would be very unsafe. For us and for your father.

I could help you.

No.

He's thinking, thinking.

The fire brigade!

I'm sorry?

You could call the fire brigade. That's what you do, isn't it? They could help you.

We'd only call the fire brigade if we couldn't get your father out any other way. So, for example, if there was an immovable obstruction.

Well, there you go.

Sir, this is not an immovable obstruction.

The son nods.

Of course. Of course.

He starts pacing back and forth. But there's no room to pace, so he's really just marching round in a tiny circle.

We're happy to move them for you.

No! No! You mustn't touch them. You MUSTN'T touch them.

Okay.

They're all in order. A very specific order. You really mustn't touch them.

That's fine. But if you don't want us to touch them, then you'll need to do it yourself. And, I'm afraid, sir, there is a time factor. So you need to make a start.

I survey the landing. A dozen stacks of newspapers line the route between the patient's bedroom and the top of the staircase – which is a separate problem all of its own. Each neatly arranged pile, I guess, consists of about a hundred broadsheet journals: over a thousand items to be moved out of the way. And right now the patient's son is still clutching the very top paper from the very first pile.

Sir? Sir?

Yes?

The papers?

The patient's son replaces the newspaper on the top of the first pile.

No.

I'm sorry?

He blinks.

It can't be done.

He turns his face away.

They're all in order. A really very quite specific order, you see. If I move them, they'll be . . . ruined.

But . . . What about your father? He's quite unwell.

He turns to face us. He pushes his glasses to the bridge of his nose.

You'll have to find another way.

We're upstairs in a house that looks like all the others from the outside. But inside it's a sinking ship. To cross the threshold, you have to force the front door back against an avalanche of textiles overflowing from the front room. The downstairs hallway is stacked floor-to-ceiling with boxes on both sides. The kitchen surfaces are crowded with tins, jars and packets of dried foods; on the floor sit crates of soft drinks shrink-wrapped in plastic, cardboard containers of cleaning products and packs of paper party crockery. The staircase is an endeavour of strange artistry. One side of it, all fourteen steps, has been commandeered as a storage platform for magazines, many still encased in cellophane: not the back issues of a treasured niche periodical, but the disposable supplements of weekend newspapers, catalogues of fleeces, china ornaments and bathroom aids, and promotional leaflets found wedged in the letterbox. These have been assembled into a precarious structure that tessellates with the steps to exploit the dead space above the stairs: the planning and dedication are at odds with its functional value, since this is a library of heft and not learning – nothing here has been read or even touched for a very long time. A glance into the bathroom reveals a similar scene: ancient scented soaps in decorative cartons misted with dust, industrial quantities of toothpaste, a multi-pack of air freshener, bottles of handwash, shower gel and bubble bath, all in bulk supply. This last item seems particularly anomalous, since the bath itself has not been filled with water any time recently; its function now is as an impromptu silo for the odd-shaped objects that cannot be stacked elsewhere. And then there's the landing and its newsprint monoliths.

This collection of rooms no longer resembles a home; it's taken on the personality of an unruly warehouse. How it came to be like this is a mystery, but it's clearly taken some commitment. It seems incredible that a middle-aged man and his elderly father have been living here so long without incident. Like many individuals outside the mainstream, they've quietly gone under the radar. But how have they cooked?

Where have they washed? What do they do to relax? Where do they go when they want a bit of *space*?

To the outside eye, this set-up looks impossible. A habitat that has abandoned its central purpose. Yet what's surprising to the seasoned paramedic is not its uniqueness but its banality; not the rarity of its domestic surrender, but the degree to which it resembles so many other household predicaments all over the city, all over the land.

While his son has been pacing about on the landing, we've helped Patrick into our carry chair in preparation for a trip to A&E. He's a tall man with a strong chin and enormous hands marbled in liver spots. I wonder what his trade was as a younger man. At eighty-four, he seems exhausted by his illness – or perhaps it's just the placidity of long-suffering. He has a fever and his legs have mislaid their power. We've changed his pyjamas and sat him on a pad because he's wet himself and there's no room to clean him up properly. We've wrapped a thin blanket and a seat belt around him and now we wheel him out into the corridor, and stop at the first stack of papers – the point where the space runs out.

What's it to be, sir? We need to get past.

The son stops pacing and turns to face his incapacitated father. He removes his glasses, pinches his temples.

What if I don't want him to go?

I'm afraid it's not your decision.

He looks close to tears.

I have to warn you, sir, that I'm going to start moving these papers now.

Would they be tears for his father, or his newsprint fortress?

I'll be as careful as I can, but I'll be moving the piles as they come and stacking them wherever I can.

Arms out, I take a step towards the first mound. I push my fingers between the sheets about a third of the way down, and drag the thick stack towards my body. There's a crackle of disintegration. The papers are yellowed and crisped at the edges from years of being grilled in the sun, and a musty odour escapes.

Just as I'm lifting the papers, the son lurches towards me, groaning like before – *Gnnnhhh!* – as if the papers are part of his body and he's in physical pain.

I stop, half-expecting to be knocked into Patrick's lap. But the son only has eyes for his journals. He forces an arm between mine, side-by-side, and takes hold of the papers and thrusts them crunchily out of my grasp and back onto the top of the pile.

I'm sorry, I'm sorry, I have to – excuse me, I'm sorry, I need to, I'm sorry – there!

He's panting. I step back, wait. He pushes the newspapers back against the wall, slides them to the left, then to the right, then left again, until he's happy they're in line.

Very quietly, in a near whisper, he speaks to the wall:

I asked you not to touch them.

It's a secret devastation. A silent internment. Nurtured and flourishing in the shadows, rampant while locked away. But once exposed to the light, suddenly tainted with shame:

I'm so sorry about the mess —
It's not usually like this —
If you'd been here last week —
We're in the middle of a clear-out —

I've come across it more times than I ever expected: it's a modern epidemic. The ex-history teacher who's made her house a storeroom for internet-bought dresses still in their plastic wrappings. The senior engineer who sleeps on the living-room floor because he can no longer get to the stairs. The retired professor whose doorframes have morphed into arches as the cobwebs have grown unopposed around the shape of her head. And the librarian who has nowhere to sit when I break the news that her mother has died in the next room, so we stand in a hallway stacked with trinkets, in a kind of limbo, with nowhere to escape to except out the front door.

How does it begin? With the careful accumulation of meaningful treasures? Tiny symbols of identity? The material keepsakes of an unfulfilled mind? Then circumstances change: a career falters, a loved one dies, and the secret cache becomes a landfill of sentiment, a barricade against loss. The stash is enriched, engorged, encumbered, and the project takes on its own momentum. Now it grows in the dark, unchallenged by outside forces, a secret wound, until the stockpile can't be touched or questioned, because if it's altered, its meaning will be lost, and its creator diminished. The possessions old and new, cherished and worthless, have become the ogre who has taken over the house, and the inhabitants are the impostors silently shuffling around the edges, knowing that something needs to be done, but unable to begin. Alteration becomes terrifying, disposal an act of bloodshed, because there's no way back, and as long as everything stays exactly as it is, where it's always been, then the emptiness will be kept at bay. Logic has gradually become stifled – behind a very normal-looking front door.

In his mid-eighties, laid low by illness, it's the patient who intervenes with a plan to make things right.

Perhaps I won't go after all . . .

I'm sorry, sir?

I think I'm going to stay at home.

Is he a peacemaker by nature, or has he become an expert at smoothing the way for his intransigent son?

Sir, you know we've advised you to come with us to hospital.

You've been very kind. Very thoughtful. But I've made up my mind. I think it's for the best.

It's the path of least resistance.

By now Patrick's daughter has arrived and squeezed past the obstructions to join the debate. She's familiar with her brother's behaviour, and seems exhausted at the prospect of having to confront it. A visit from the GP gets her vote: it sidesteps the inevitable clash and still gets her father seen. But she knows it's just postponing the inevitable.

We explain our concerns from top to bottom once again. We make it clear that what matters is Patrick's wellbeing, and the clutter in the house should not be part of the decision process. Of course it is, on some level, and probably always has been. This dynamic may be strange and new to us, but Patrick has been wrestling with it for years.

In the end it's his decision, and he's not feeling strong enough to tackle the problem in his current state. Reluctantly, we put him back in his room and leave the daughter to watch over him. We arrange for the doctor to call, possibly visit, and he or she will prescribe some antibiotics, and hopefully Patrick will recover. The daughter says she'll visit to check, and if Dad deteriorates she'll call again. And whether it's tomorrow or two years from now, one day a crew will return, and this time Patrick will have to go to hospital, and the crew will still have a house full of obstacles and their middle-aged curator to contend with, before they even get to the top of those stairs.

XI

As I step into the room I can see we're not required.

The first responder is already on scene: he's sat on a low chair, legs crossed, hands in his pockets. The patient's talking on her mobile. Her friend's boiling the kettle. Even the air in the room is relaxed.

This is what happens once the initial panic has been dealt with: a kind of relieved languor descends; the adjustment back to reality. By the time the door has closed behind us, my brain has already switched into coasting mode.

We're in the medical room at a secondary school. A teacher has fainted, then recovered. Our colleague's done what needs to be done, but the patient now feels better and doesn't want to go to A&E. We'll have a little chat, make a few jokes, check the red flags, then leave the patient with some paperwork as a souvenir. If we happen to get offered a cup of tea in the process, well, it would be rude to say no.

I'm afraid we don't have any biscuits.

No biscuits? What kind of school is this?

Someone knocks and says there's a second patient. Can we

take a look? The tea's just finished brewing: hopefully another 'non-convey'. Then a girl is brought in on the school wheel-chair and it's a swerve in the road, an electric shock, a blast of cold air.

It takes about three seconds to realise. Time to restart the brain. The teacher is already a distant memory. This is our patient. This is why we're here. And we need to get moving.

You might assume the burden of my new responsibilities as a paramedic had been apparent from the start. But the truth is they had crept up on me, like a particularly stealthy charity mugger, and I think it was better that way: I was far happier responding to the needs of patients in the heat of the moment than in giving too much thought to the notion that from time to time someone's life might be in my hands.

I've already explained how I slipped into the job when no one was looking, like an accidental tourist, all the time wait-ing for a human-resources sentinel to step into my path with a raised arm and a resolute shake of the head. A similar bash-fulness characterised my progress through the ranks once I was on board: I shuffled inconspicuously from the wide-eyed ignorance of a trainee to the awed apprehensions of a junior clinician. Then, in what felt like the blink of an eye, I was suddenly faced with the terrifying prospect of becoming the senior crew member – the one with all the hard-earned wis-dom and local coffee shop knowledge, the one your crewmate turns to anxiously when a rogue rhythm appears on the ECG screen or the patient does something that wasn't covered in the training manual.

The accompanying fears were based less on the prospect of treating patients who were critically ill or seriously injured, and more on the possibility that people could have things wrong with them that were beyond my range – what I thought of as the limitless world of potential biological catastrophe. It seemed entirely feasible that patients could be drastically unwell without me even noticing – because how could I ever know all the possible things that might go wrong with the most complex organism in the world? How could anyone? I had been taught about the respiratory system, the circulatory system, heart attacks, trauma, strokes and more. But what about all those conditions they hadn't had time to tell me about? Was it possible that some day one of those rarer pathologies would play out disastrously in front of my eyes without me even realising?

She looks like she's breathing through a straw. Fast, yes, but it's not the speed. The *work* is the tell. The effort. Sitting in a chair, arched forward, eyes wide, she is pure mechanics: a relentless athlete of respiration. Nothing else counts. Right now, shifting a cupful of air from one place to another is her body's sole concern.

Her name is Anna. Sixteen and asthmatic. Been out on the games field. In a flash come over short of breath. Used her inhaler to no effect. A paper hat in a rainstorm.

I feel her wrist, scan her face. Her eyes are bright with a terror she has no breath to verbalise. My colleague grabs a nebuliser. This is the basic, animal fear. Running out of air. Like claustrophobia – but inside the body. I pull out my stethoscope and listen to her chest. There's a wheeze, yes, but what concerns me is the expansion of her ribs. Each time she breathes, they lift and then sink as if they're straining against the skin that surrounds them. An extravagant movement: a tiny return.

My crewmate looks up from the oxygen bag.

Atrovent as well?

Absolutely.

She adds the drugs to the chamber, connects the tubing, straps on the mask. The oxygen blasts the liquid into a mist, to be dragged down into Anna's lungs.

Let's get her out to the truck. Then hydrocortisone. Adrenaline. And we'll put in a call.

Calling 999 is simple – as it should be. No one wants to be looking up a number when their child's having a convulsion, or scrabbling around for their car keys when their colleague's collapsed on the floor. Calling for help wouldn't be calling for help if you needed to be on top of your game to do it.

What happens next? Someone answers your call. They confirm your address and put you in the system. Ask what's happened. Find out what's wrong. The call is categorised: now you're one of the 'calls holding' – a string of numbers, a coloured dot on a map. You exist – or you will do as soon as we have someone available to send. Now your status depends on the route you've taken through the flowchart; your identity is the result of how closely you match a set of criteria.

Someone else looks at the call and, so long as one's available, an ambulance is dispatched. Sometimes a car, or a bike – if they think the patient will benefit from some early intervention. Very occasionally a helicopter. The crew receives the job. They start making their way. They're given a brief summary of what's been reported, which may or may not be accurate. By the time they arrive, they have a sense of what to expect and are ready to go.

From time to time, though, no call is needed. Just occasionally a patient finds there's already a crew at hand – across the road, outside the door, in a room down the hall. These jobs that crews come upon coincidentally are sometimes referred to as 'running calls':

What's that yellow thing outside?

A Morrison's van?

No. You won't believe this. It's an ambulance.

Not all running calls are dire emergencies, of course; many occur as a kind of Pavlovian response to seeing something big and yellow – like beginning to salivate as you pass the donuts in Tesco, or needing a pee by a waterfall – and turn out to have a very thin connection to the word *emergency*. But every once in a while, a genuinely time-critical patient, such as Anna today, gets very lucky indeed. In these cases, the time it takes to call 999 and receive a response might make all the difference in the world.

For the ambulance crew, these 'right place, right time' jobs demand an abrupt change of pace. There's been no warning, no preparation. No psychological separation between the event and the response to it. When an emergency lands in a crew's lap unannounced, it requires a more instinctive response. If the patient's sick, this is when the crew needs to be on their game. One moment they're polishing their haloes and dunking a chocolate Hobnob, the next someone's life is on the line.

Anna is sat up straight on the trolley bed, travelling backwards at speed, her eyes silently pleading, her breathing no calmer, her shoulders lifting, falling, lifting, falling.

The in-breath is an act of willpower, as if she's trying to ration herself. Her body wants to gulp more air but there's nowhere to put it; she can't get it back out. She's a stopped-up bellows, a bottleneck. Not a gasp but a whisper. As she exhales, her lips form the tiny O of someone blowing on a hot drink with a bus to catch. Only there's more at stake than being late for work. As soon as one breath is achieved, she embarks on the next. There's neither intermission nor rest.

Hospital is five miles away but we're on the way and moving fast. I'm in the back, attaching equipment, fetching drugs, chatting to the patient with all the calmness I can muster. But mostly keeping busy trying to stay on my feet. My crewmate keeps braking for the traffic, accelerating away from it, braking again. I pitch forward, lurch back, grab at the bars above my head like a sailor in a storm. I set my feet wide apart, shout through to remind my colleague I'm upright and would like to stay that way, but I'm starting to feel like a yoyo.

There's a balance to be struck here. Velocity is the name of the game – that's what all those lights and sirens are for. But effective treatment is disrupted by haste; it comes with composure and clarity of thought. Deep breath: steady hands. We want to get this patient to A&E without delay, but the journey time is the golden window of intervention, the opportunity that a blind rush would waste. There are things that can be done, must be done – things that might change the outcome – along the way.

Anna's body is confused. It's attacking itself. It's detected something hostile in the system, but the responses are making things worse. Her airways have gone into a kind of spasm, as if they've got stage-fright and have forgotten their lines; they're closing in on themselves, rigid with shame at their own failure, and she can't move the air she needs. In the emergency hierarchy, this is pretty much the top of the tree: she's on the precipice.

It's a vicious circle. Since the passages to Anna's lungs are squeezed, she has to work harder to drag the oxygen in and push it back out – but that very effort means she needs more of the stuff. We're giving her oxygen, so the air she's breathing is rich in what she needs. But it's not fixing the underlying malfunction; it's just filling her chest up with air.

I've replenished the medicine in the mask. This should act on the spasm – but it's not helped yet. Another drug we've given should open up the airways – no sign so far. Before we left we gave her a small shot of adrenaline – which has made no change up until now. I'll give her some more in a moment.

These drugs should be making Anna better, but so far nothing's improved.

There's one more medicine I need to give. I'd considered injecting the muscle, but I want to get it in the vein where it can work faster. This means a cannula on the move in the back of a moving truck.

Anna, I need to put a little needle in your arm. There's another medicine and it needs to go in your vein. Okay?

She nods.

We really should stop and do this at the side of the road – this is the Right Thing to Do – but I don't want the delay. The traffic is stacked today and the drivers seem especially reluctant to surrender the road. All the vehicles we've just overtaken will come back past and we'll have to do it all over again. If I keep a steady hand, and an eye on the road, I can get the needle in while we're weaving through the queue at the lights.

I kneel beside the trolley, tie the tourniquet around Anna's upper arm, tap and clean the small blue ridge that appears in her flesh. I glance out to check we're not about to pull away or slam on the anchors, line up the cannula and slide the needle into the skin like a plane touching down. A tiny drop of blood pops into the chamber. I retract the needle and advance the plastic, remove the sharp and fix the cap. I secure the cannula and push a small flush of salt water. This all sounds smooth, painless, calm. If only that were the case.

I draw up the steroid, push it in through the cannula, as slowly as I can bear, followed by more salty water. I give another shot of adrenaline in the muscle and check the medicine in the mask. I look out of the window to see where we are. Maybe five minutes to go. Anna's had all the medicine she can have; there's nothing left for me to give.

Since the power of my ignorance seemed to reside in its limitlessness, it seemed the only logical solution was to turn around and look the other way. Not to bury my head in the sand exactly, but rather to redirect my attention, to simplify, in effect to triage myself. Rather than worry about the vast imaginarium of alternative possible pathologies, I focused on what I could and should do in any given situation and put the rest to one side: recognising when there was a problem, giving the treatment within my remit, and referring upwards when something fell beyond. The moment I began to feel less overwhelmed was when I realised that in any given scenario, my task could be distilled down to three simple questions. If I could answer those questions, and respond appropriately, I was most of the way there.

The second of these questions came to me first, because it was the oldest, from a time long ago, when the focus of ambulance work was transport – removing patients from harm and taking them to a place of safety and repair – and the principal skill was recognising the urgency of transfer. The third question came next, a result of the growing arsenal of emergency treatments available within the ambulance itself. And the first question to answer, ironically, was the newest of the three, a product of the recent changes in emergency triage, and the proliferation of non-emergency 999 calls that would never go near A&E. The questions were as follows:

1. *Does the patient need to go to hospital?*
2. *If so, how quickly does the patient need to get there?*
3. *What can be done for them on the way?*

This was my route to simplicity and conviction. As a friend of mine used to say, it's not rocket surgery.

For our original patient, our fainting teacher, the first question was answered with a no, and that was the end of the story: our first responder was left to dot the Is and cross the Ts. But in Anna's case, the answers were more involved: 1. yes; 2. as quickly as possible; and 3. oxygen, appropriate escalating drugs protocol and, potentially, bag-valve resuscitation if things did not improve. Anything further was beyond my reach.

As gently as I can, I encourage Anna to slow her breathing down. This is the last thing she wants to hear. Of course it is. Everyone I meet at work breathes fast, but this is not panic, or not just panic. This is exhaustion, and the very real fear that she's running out of air. This would make anyone panic. But panicked breathing is ineffective breathing. It's not just air, but energy she's running out of. If this goes on much longer, I might have to start ventilating the patient myself.

I find a bag-valve mask and set it up. It looks like a see-through rugby ball attached to a padded face mask, and it's for pushing oxygen into lungs that have stopped drawing air in themselves. It is not what I had in mind when I strolled into the medical room and saw the kettle boiling and my colleague with his feet up. I'm just about to switch the mask when I'm thrown off to the side and into the passenger seat at the back of the truck. Good. This means we're circling the roundabout near the hospital.

And it's then that I notice a change. It's Anna's breathing. It's slowing down. And not just slowing. Calming. Relaxing. Returning to something more normal. The steroid. The cortico-glorious-magical-steroid.

Within seconds we're at the A&E. We wheel Anna into resus and she shuffles onto the hospital bed. I give my handover off the top of my head to the waiting team – what was wrong, what we found, what we did, how it helped. I'm a little short of breath myself. A little warm and drained after being thrown about the back of the ambulance with a young girl's fate on my mind. Unclear on the history. Unable to recall the exact dose of the drugs.

In contrast, the doctor stands and listens like he's contemplating a sunset over the Tuscan hills. He could look no more relaxed if he were wearing cargo shorts and sipping Chianti. It's not that he's rude. It's just that he seems to be struggling to match what I'm telling him about Anna's really quite perilous initial presentation with the patient we've put in front of him. Could it be that we've transported the wrong girl?

The problem is, Anna suddenly looks rather well. Her breathing has relaxed. Her observations are approaching normal. She no longer looks like she's about to drop.

Except, I realise, as I head back out to the truck and spot myself reflected in the automatic resus doors, flushed and sweaty, this is not a problem. This is, of course, the very opposite of a problem. The doctor's dismissiveness, in fact, has made me inordinately happy. It's not a criticism; it's a ringing endorsement. The clearest proof that today my colleague and I have had the chance to do our job.

XII

The first encounter is the moment of truth. When we walk through the door and see the patient for the first time: this is the instant of revelation, the confirmation or rejection of what we've been told in advance; the moment we know what kind of job it will be. This is when the emergency goes live.

Until that moment, the patient is an abstract. An unconfirmed rumour. A job we could be cancelled off before arrival. An age, a gender, a flowchart diagnosis, a misspelt name on a screen. An exaggeration, a mix-up, a panic, a rumour.

But in that first informative glimpse, potential is wiped out by reality; assumptions are brushed aside by the palpable substance of a human form. There's an influx of messages – posture, alertness, skin colour, tone, responsiveness, effort, fatigue – a complex chorus of tiny assessments that validate or challenge the claims that have been made. As the details resolve into a logical ensemble, one of two things happens: either the brain relaxes to standby – or the adrenaline kicks in.

*

The patient's mother leads us up the broken stairs. Our boots beat a rhythm on the bare wood. It's not a dirty house: it just boasts of little care. The walls are dark with life-grime and shiny with years of friction at elbow height, as if it's never occurred to anyone to add another coat of paint. The carpet has been removed but never replaced. The smoke alarm issues the customary bleep.

The patient's in the front bedroom, bent forward in a low chair in front of the window. It's a bright day, and light streams through the blinds across his shoulders and onto his knees. He looks up as we enter, his shaven head a glossy silhouette.

And this is the moment of truth.

When the job was dispatched, we were given the address and the following description:

38-YEAR-OLD MALE, VOMITING BLOOD
[DANGEROUS HAEMORRHAGE; CATEGORY 2]

A man in his thirties who's apparently vomiting blood. Likelihood? A stomach bug, D&V for a couple of days? Spotted some pink streaks amid the regurgitated food? Asked by the call-taker if there's blood in his vomit, he's replied *yes*, and it's become a life-threatening call.

I approach the patient and spin the blind to block out the glare. Introductions are made; I take the patient's wrist.

You've been vomiting, Gavin?

I thought it would've stopped, but it's just got worse.

How long's it been going on?

This time? A week.

You've had it before?
Lots of times. When I've been drinking.
Alcohol?
He nods.
Are you alcohol dependent, Gavin?
He nods.

Gavin is thin, gaunt. The pulse at his wrist is rapid. His eyes are withdrawn into their orbits. His shoulders rise and fall with each breath. He looks sapped. Then there's his skin. It's pale, moist, waxy, insipid. It looks . . . what? Artificial. It reminds me of the candles on my bathroom window sill, their glossy sheen beaded with moisture after a day in the sun.

My crewmate and I give each other the look. A tiny twitch of the eyebrows mirrored back and forth: let's not hang around.

Any blood in the vomit? Any bile?
The last few days it's been blood.
Pure blood? Or streaks?
He shakes his head.
Bright red.
How much d'you think?
A lot.
How many times?
This morning, every half an hour.
Gavin, do you feel faint?
I'm sorry for swearing.
How d'you mean?
I feel like shit.

This short conversation has worn Gavin out. My crewmate turns to fetch the chair, then has a thought.

Do you want your cannula roll?

Good idea.

We help Gavin into the chair. He resists the strap, says it makes him feel trapped, but he knows he's too weak to walk.

Try not to grab out, Gavin. Keep your hands in your lap, okay?

We wheel him to the stairs, oxygen mask on his face, IV cannula in his arm, and carry him down, grateful that he's so skinny. As we roll to the front door and lift him over the threshold, he suddenly grabs the doorframe and drags himself back.

Wait!

He's half-in and half-out of the house, one paramedic behind him in the hallway, the other at his feet, outside. He looks anxiously around.

What is it, Gavin?

Where are my trainers?

He pulls off the oxygen mask, tries to stand up.

Your trainers?

I need my trainers.

You're wearing them, Gavin.

I need my trainers.

You've got your trainers on.

Not these. Where have they gone? Mum! Can you get me my trainers?

Wait, wait, wait. Just relax. What's going on, Gavin? What's wrong with these ones?

He's trying to undo the buckle on the strap. Another glance between the two crewmates.

Okay, Gavin. Let's stay nice and calm. Let's leave the strap there. We don't want you to fall. You know, I think these ones are fine. They'll only take them off at the hospital.

But he's pulling at the laces.

I'm not going.

Sorry?

I want my trainers.

Fine. Okay. We'll get your trainers. Will they be down here? Or up in your room?

I don't know! Mum!

What is it?

I need my trainers. I think they're in my room.

His mother's steps echo on the stairs.

I tell you what, Gavin, why don't we get you settled on the ambulance and your mum can bring them out in a moment?

But Gavin puts out his arms to the doorframe again and, gulping his breaths, quietly murmurs:

I'm not going out there . . . without my trainers on.

The longer he delays, the more concerned we become – and the sooner we want to get going. This might be a psychological hurdle – perhaps Gavin rarely leaves the house and is panicking at the prospect. But we both suspect a physiological reason – serious haemorrhage and a confused, oxygen-deprived brain. If he's been vomiting fresh, frank blood, there's a good chance he has varices and unchecked bleeding in his oesophagus, as a result of his drinking. His rapid breathing and pallor, his distress and his evident

124

weakness, all suggest that he's already lost a significant quantity of blood.

The endgame is getting Gavin outside and on his way to A&E. We could drag the chair with him kicking and screaming. We could give him fluids here on the doorstep. But if the clues are to be trusted, he needs hospital treatment, soon.

But here's where the balance has to be struck. This is real-world patient management, a long way from a clinical cubicle, and if getting Gavin outside safely means taking the time to change his shoes for him, then that's what we'll do.

I had completed my last spell of training and was now working with the word PARAMEDIC inscribed across each shoulder. This was a double-edged sword: an endorsement and an obligation. On the one hand, I felt I'd earned my stripes and my sea legs. On the other, I now knew the buck stopped with me.

There's often a misunderstanding about the term *paramedic* and its alternatives. In ambulance work, there are paramedics and there are non-paramedics – technicians, assistants, practitioners; a variety of names for basically the same thing.

The key message is that essentially everyone does the same job. If an emergency ambulance comes to your door, you might get a double-medic crew, but it's also possible you'll get a crew of two non-paramedics.

It would be a mistake to assume that a non-paramedic is somehow less proficient; often technicians have done many years in the job and are exactly the people you want around you in a crisis. In my early days as a medic, I frequently sought advice and reassurance from my more experienced non-medic crewmates. I still do it now.

The main distinction is that paramedics have a few extra skills at their disposal, and carry a few flashier drugs: more options for pain management, medicines for fits and allergies and so on. So in a crisis, technicians are more likely to head for hospital, whereas a paramedic might take a bit of time to offer treatment on scene.

Where Gavin was concerned, my status as a medic meant I could put a needle in his vein and give him some fluids, which would be helpful but far from decisive. I could also give him an anti-sickness drug, but I chose not to because he hadn't vomited with us, and I felt that right now we had bigger fish to fry. There was nothing I could do about his internal haemorrhage, so the main treatment we could give him was diesel. No matter what the clinical grade, the key skill here was the same as ever: identifying a 'big sick' patient and facilitating a rapid transfer to definitive care.

Once we've got Gavin on the bed, my crewmate and I glide around each other, swooping towards him and away again, reconnecting oxygen, hooking up equipment, running up fluids, lifting his legs. This kind of thing is a fleet-footed *pas de deux* in a tiny space – efficient and seamless if the crewmates know and trust each other; laboured and clumsy if not.

Gavin's mother sits hunched in the corner seat, silent and unobtrusive in the manner of family members who can read the signs. Ambulance crews regularly reassure families with the words, 'As long as we're relaxed, you should be relaxed.'

The counterpart is that when crews drop the chit-chat and start working quickly and purposefully, the contrary implications are clear.

Within a few minutes we've done what we can on scene and are ready to go. We pass the details over the radio, so the controller can pre-alert the hospital. My crewmate jumps in the front, on go the blue lights, we spin around and head off.

Since we've laid Gavin on the bed, his blood pressure has improved. His breathing seems less laboured with the oxygen. He's more relaxed since he changed his shoes. We're close to the hospital. Within ten minutes he'll be in resus and receiving the care he needs.

Then, within a minute of leaving scene, Gavin sits up. He looks around as if he's been startled from a dream, peers with confusion at all the apparatus, his mother in the corner, the paramedic by his side.

Gavin? You okay? You're in an ambulance, Gavin. Those noises are just the sirens. We're going round the traffic. We'll be at hospital soon. Sit back, Gavin. Just relax.

But Gavin is not relaxing, he's trying to stand up. He swings his legs off the trolley, but they're obstructed by the bar along the side of the bed, which he pulls at, thinking he can detach it. It's as if he has no memory of how he got here. He looks down at his feet and begins kicking one shoe against the other, toe against heel. One of the trainers he was so insistent about somersaults off across the ambulance; his mother picks it up. Then the blood-pressure cuff inflates: he looks at his left arm, reaches for the Velcro and yanks it off. The cuff springs back towards the monitor, getting caught in the fluid line.

Gavin, Gavin. Try to sit still. Let's put your legs back up on the bed.

I reach out to Gavin but my arm is pushed away. Gavin pulls off the oxygen mask as if in an act of self-defence. He takes deep, gasping breaths. He stares at me, facing down his tormentor. His arms pull at the wires. He's sweating profusely and the sticky pads have come loose. The wires add to the tangle of leads around his IV line.

My crewmate behind the wheel can sense the threat of chaos:

Everything okay back there?

We've become a bit agitated.

Then, just as we swerve, Gavin's mum undoes her belt and stands to reach out to her son.

No, no, no. Sorry, madam. You need to sit down. Please.

I usher her back to her seat.

We don't want you to fall.

Gavin pulls the probe off his finger and grabs the fluid line running down to his arm.

Gavin! Gavin!

He twirls the clear tube around his hand and yanks it out of his arm. It pings across the ambulance, spraying salty water across the bed and floor. Then blood begins to flow from the vein, running off the crook of his arm and seeping into the bed sheet.

In one move I stand, scoop Gavin's legs up, dump them back onto the bed, grab the end of the belt and yank it tight across Gavin's thighs, then shove him back to a lying position, an act he has no strength to resist. I tug a wad of blue roll from the dispenser and press it against the haemorrhaging vein with my left hand: with my right at full stretch I open one of the eye-level cupboards, dragging out the pouch of dressings, gripping the bag between my arm and my ribs to open the zip one-handed, so that the dressings spill out onto the bed and the floor, then grab one at random, tearing the packaging and swapping it in for the sodden blue roll, tying it roughly but tightly in place on his arm. From up front, the driver asks:

Do you want me to stop?

How far away are we?

Two minutes.

Keep going.

I turn off the fluids, take a breath and a step back, holding onto the ceiling bar as we round a wide bend.

Gavin's eyes are closed now, as if he's withdrawn into some private chamber, hugging his knees in the terrified dark. Does he have a sense of how unwell he is? He's pulled all the monitoring off, but no technology is needed to see what's going on. His breathing has become shallow, his pulse weak. Any colour that had returned has disappeared again. Gavin's body is making one last desperate effort of self-preservation. His organs are burning the last of their reserves in an attempt to save the ensemble, before they collapse for ever.

I grab the tangle of wires and wrench it out of the way – they're no use now. I take a bag-valve mask from the cupboard and connect it to the oxygen. I lay Gavin's head flat and cup the mask over his mouth and nose, lift his jaw to make a seal and begin to squeeze slow, measured breaths of pure oxygen into Gavin's chest, still watching and feeling for a pulse. If

Gavin's mother didn't grasp the seriousness before, she surely does now.

We pull into the ambulance bay, lower the back, wheel the trolley onto the tail-lift and off again at ground level, and push Gavin into the resus room, all the while supporting his breathing. He's not fighting us now.

The doctor has her own moment of truth when she spots the bag-valve mask and seamlessly changes gear, suddenly barking orders, calling for an anaesthetist, taking handover as she initiates treatment. She's not afraid to raise her voice when things don't happen as she expects them to, and for a few minutes of the initial clamour we remain involved in Gavin's care, before stepping aside and leaving him in their hands.

My final deed will be to register Gavin at reception, but I don't even have a surname – these things can slip through the net in a dynamic emergency – so I head to the relatives' room to find his mum. Her imploring eyes look up as I enter, and for a moment they flicker with hope, but then it seems to get washed away in the blinked-back salt water. I do my best to answer her questions, but I have limited information and can't say too much because I'm no longer responsible for Gavin's care.

I can't give her the one reply she wants, so I leave her waiting in a windowless room, her son's one trainer on the low table in front of her.

XIII

Ambulance crews are a cantankerous breed. Easily irked, proudly rebellious and expertly grumpy, we enjoy nothing more than getting stuck into a really wholesome, satisfying moan. Patients, management, colleagues, dispatchers: all themes are welcome. And not without purpose: as a way of fostering solidarity among peers, moaning is surely just as effective as paint-balling or raft-building. Plus, you can eat a donut while you're doing it.

It's often said the NHS runs on the goodwill of its staff. If its ambulance services are anything to go by, you might say it's powered to an even greater degree by the inexhaustible fuel of communal complaint.

Of course, grumbling with workmates is one of the great unifying pleasures of any job, but when you're on a twelve-hour shift, working your way through a list of shared frustrations can really make the time fly. Carping about the nonsense calls that require none of your expertise, then whining about the proper jobs that involve some actual work; condemning management for being out of touch with frontline staff, before scoffing at their attempts to engage us in the process of change: there's really so much to choose from. Happily, the contradictions do nothing to stem the energising torrent of frustration that keeps weary crews going at two a.m.

There are plenty of subjects that lend themselves to this soothing refrain. For some, the great antagonist is the obstructive driving of other road users: the non-puller-overs, the wave-you-throughers, the under-takers and the tail-gaters. For others, it's the lack of support from superiors which provides the most persistent wound. But, if there were a hierarchy of grievance, there would surely be one undisputed champion: the perennial discrepancy between the intended purpose of emergency resources and the casual reality of the calls we actually attend. In other words: the misuse of the service.

It's possible that when I first put on my green combats, I was suffering from delusions of grandeur about how my days were going to take shape. Delivering babies in the frozen aisle of Asda, I thought. Cannulating patients under a bus in the pouring rain. Defibrillating trembling hearts on a train platform. Wrestling drunks. And lots and lots of car crashes. Not quite rock and roll, but a long way from fiddling with the formula functions in Excel.

It didn't take me long to be disabused. The truth soon became apparent: I was going to spend a lot of my time telling people how to take paracetamol.

They say if you go tiger-hunting, don't be surprised when you come across a tiger. Ambulance crews deal with genuine emergencies. Obviously they do, because that's why the job exists. Right now there'll be a crew somewhere dealing with each of the gory dramas you can imagine. Stemming the flow. Opening the airway. Cutting the cord. Pushing rhythmically on the chest. Rushing to hospital. But there'll be many more who went tiger-hunting and found rabbits: who are, at this very moment, calmly reassuring a distressed patient that things are not as bad as they seem. Bringing some realism to bear on someone's temporary crisis. Untangling the threads of a problem to put things into perspective. Because, in the back of the ambulance, with all that equipment and those lights and sirens and emergency drugs, the medicine we dispense most of is common sense.

And paracetamol. Plenty of paracetamol.

Which might play out as follows:

Where does it hurt?

Everywhere!

How long have you been unwell?

Two days.

You're running a fever. Have you taken any painkillers?

Paracetamol.

When did you take it?

It didn't work.

When did you take it?

After I got up.

Okay. What time was that?

Eleven o'clock.

This morning?

Yesterday.

You haven't taken any since yesterday morning?

I keep my voice soft: this is not an accusation. But I sense that the patient doesn't like where this is going. She's wondering why the man in green keeps going on about paracetamol. He seems a bit obsessed. She's wondering why we're not already on the way to hospital. She's wondering if I'm a real paramedic. She starts looking at my uniform suspiciously: it doesn't seem to be very well ironed.

It didn't work.

Okay. So you can definitely take some more now. How many did you take?

One.

Right. You could have taken two.

Two?

Two.

At the same time?

At the same time.

I normally only take one.

That's why it's not working.

Haven't you got anything stronger?

What we have here is a disparity. The patient feels awful. She probably doesn't think she's dying, but she does think she's just about as ill as any human has ever been, and it's going to take some pretty high-end gear to get her back on her feet. Possibly something involving needles. Definitely something with a really long name. I, on the other hand, suspect she has a viral fever, which some rest, fluids and painkillers will probably knock on the head in a couple of days.

Let's take two of these now and see how we go.

But isn't it dangerous? To take too much?

Too much would be more than eight tablets in one day. You've taken one tablet in two days.

I don't want to get addicted.

You won't get addicted.

But will it work?

How do you mean?

Will it get rid of it?

It won't get rid of the infection, if that's what it is. But it will help with the pain, and it will help with the fever, which will make you feel better.

What's the point in taking it then?

It will help you feel better. While your body fights the illness.

I want the tablet that gets rid of the illness. Give me that tablet.

I don't have that tablet.

Why not?

We don't carry antibiotics. And you probably don't need them.

So the tablets you want me to take —

Paracetamol.

— They're just going to hide the problem.

Not exactly.

I'll feel better but I'll still be ill.

Have I got the energy to tackle this one now? The one about painkillers masking pain. I decide this is a battle for another day. Right now I'm steeling myself for the every-four-hours-you-can-take-two-more-tablets conversation. And I haven't even mentioned the word *ibuprofen* yet . . .

Don't you want to feel better?

No.

No?

135

I want to get better.

Okay. I think you've got a fairly simple infection. You're young and healthy and your observations are normal. You have no what we call red flags. You've got a high temperature because your body is fighting off the illness. That's why you feel rough. That's why you're exhausted. It's going to take a bit of time for your body to overcome it, but it should do so in a few days. If you keep yourself cool, drink plenty of water, take regular paracetamol, then you won't feel so ill while your body's doing what it needs to do.

If you can't make me better, I want to go to hospital so they can make me better.

You're welcome to go to hospital if you want to. But you don't really need to. And there'll be a long wait. And you'll be sat in a waiting room with lots of other ill people. And I doubt they'll give you what you want.

So what do you suggest?

I suggest you turn the heating off and open a window. Take away a couple of those duvets. Drink plenty of water.

I don't drink water.

Or some other fluids. And take regular paracetamol. Regularly. So that's two tablets, every four to six hours. Okay? So we'll take two now, and you can take two more in four hours' time.

Four hours?

Yep.

I can take them again?

This is not secret information. This is printed on the back of the packet.

So what time?

Well, it's quarter to midnight now. So, if you're still awake at quarter to four, you can take two more.

Yeah, but what if I'm asleep?

Then it won't matter. You can take some when you wake up. And then, four hours after that, you can take two more. As long as you don't take more than eight tablets in twenty-four hours, you can have them every four to six hours.

It sounds confusing. Can you write it down for me?

It's written on the back of the box.

I know, but when you're ill it's hard to read.

I take a deep breath.

Sure. I'll write it down.

I write down the dose instructions on a piece of paper, wondering how to make my writing clearer than the printing on the packet. I pop two tablets from the strip and hold them out. The patient looks at the tablets but doesn't take them. Are they real? There's a tiny part of her that still believes I'm a sales rep from a drugs company.

You're sure it will work?

I'm sure it will help.

And you want me to take both of them?

Boom. This is it. This is the question.

I always thought I was a patient man, but lately two recurring episodes are causing me to doubt myself. One is when I try to get my kids out of the house for the school run. The other is when someone utters the words, *You want me to take them both?*

I've been through an approximation of this conversation seven or eight times this week, and I've kept my cool so far. But right now I want to punch myself in the face. Blow the world's biggest raspberry. Shake the patient by the shoulders.

Scrawl my resignation on the wall in tomato ketchup. *You want me to take two?* No! I don't care if you take two, or one, or none. You called me with a problem, an emergency problem. And I'm giving you a solution. A simple solution you had at your fingertips the whole time. You are not doing me a favour. I do *not* want you to take them both. You can do whatever you want . . .

Deep breath. Stop complaining. It's a job, is it not, and an easy one at that? This lady's simply out of her depth. She just wants to be told everything's okay by someone she can trust. Is it her fault she's the third patient in a row who doesn't know how to cope with a fever? The fifth person this week who can dial 999 but doesn't believe in taking tablets? The thing is, this is supposed to be the job where you never know what's coming next. Right now it's pretty easy to guess.

All occupations are encumbered by predictability, I tell myself. It would be an inefficient workman who learnt a fresh skill every day but never used any of them twice. So is this mere frustration with the banalities of a daily routine? Perhaps. But what's galling about this encounter is not its resemblance to so many of its predecessors; it's the sense of tacit acquiescence. The feeling that it's pointless getting annoyed by such non-emergencies, because the future holds a hundred identical patients and any indignation will only make dealing with them harder, so why bother? Besides, on some level it's their imposture in the emergency system that keeps us all employed. Complaining about it serves about as much purpose as shouting into a well.

I know all this. And yet the well retains a strange allure:

it has excellent acoustics and a soothing echo. Perfect for a night shift alone in a car.

Imagine an enthusiastic graphic designer, freshly graduated and arriving for her first day at a leading design agency. She's given a colouring book and some felt tips.

What's this?

She's confused. But her boss beams with fervour:

Colouring! Make sure you do a good job! We're counting on you!

But . . . I thought I'd be doing . . . well, design?

She stares at the stationery in her hands.

You will! From time to time. Maybe once or twice a week. But mainly, we'd like you to do colouring in! Also, dot-to-dots. Do you like puzzles? Great!

The boss grins encouragingly.

Now, we want you to be really neat. Make sure you stay within the lines . . .

An endless roster of non-emergency calls is not just demoralising for clinicians; it's also enormously inefficient. It puts unsustainable pressure on ambulance services because there's too much work for the available resources, and the services are failing, and the sickest patients are waiting, not because people are having more heart attacks or serious accidents, but because of the exponential increase in calls to the sort of minor problems that can be managed at home. This discrepancy is gradually bringing down the walls from the inside. It leads to a workforce deskilled in its supposed speciality, and contributes to a sense of burnout in road staff (even if it does give them something to moan about through the small hours).

Most significantly, though, this incongruity means that patients with genuine emergencies often receive a delayed response, and that their care suffers as a result. Fundamentally, it's an abuse of a system set up for the common good.

People suffering a time-critical medical emergency should be able to call for help and be confident they'll receive a timely response from clinicians skilled in giving treatment and with plenty of diesel and some lights and sirens.

People suffering with a high temperature should open a window, drink plenty of water and, if they want to feel better, take two – yes, two – paracetamol.

The patient stares expectantly at me, the man in green. My face shows no sign of murderous intent. I gulp and sigh and think about the aroma of freshly brewed coffee. All things must end. I have a pack of custard creams waiting in my car. And some lukewarm tea. This woman only wants some reassurance and a bit of advice.

I smile warmly.

Yes, I do want you to take two. Let's give it a try, shall we? Let me get you some water.

XIV

The city's been hot and sticky and unforgiving for a fortnight. The grass in the parks is scorched to stubble; there's dust in the air and not a cloud in the sky. Every window that opens has been pushed wide to its limit, but there's no breeze and the heat just keeps coming – from the air, from the earth, from the buildings and pavements and roads and vehicles, from the fridges and freezers and flat-screen TVs and even the fans, and from inside the walls. No one's been sleeping, and everyone can hear everyone else's business, their bickering and bawling, their apologies and reconciliations, their gossiping and gloating and sickly affections, and especially their music, their terrible, terrible music.

Of course the call rate's high. Not just the drinking in the parks and the tempers running short and the muggy evening police jobs: assaults, stabbings, mental health. Chronic conditions made worse by the heat. Asthmatics who haven't had an attack for years. Diabetics with low sugar. The elderly dehydrated. Infants unable to sleep. Teenagers fainting before their exams. A population of aliens crammed together, waiting for the storm to break.

I'm on a late shift on a car, covering the busiest part of the day, overlapping the transition between days and nights. The idea is that a non-transporting vehicle is more likely to be available, so when a high-category call comes in the responder can get there more quickly – and meet the all-important response times.

This is a recent undertaking for me, and the reality is still hitting home. Working on the car means working alone, and this brings a whole new brand of terror. It's like being a rookie all over again. There's no one to turn to for a word of advice – or even a reassuring shrug of shared perplexity. There's no one to send outside for the chair when all else fails – and no chair outside to send for, even if there was. There's no way of leaving for the sanctuary of hospital, because I'm on a non-transporting vehicle. On an FRU, you're stuck on scene, doing what you can with what you've got, often in a cluttered, or chaotic, or hostile environment, until someone comes and rescues you.

Suddenly everything I'm sent to sounds incredibly serious – as if my move has corrected all the problems with the triage system and catastrophe awaits me at every turn. Of course I'm forgetting that these are the same jobs as before – I'm just going to them in a different guise.

I'm dispatched to a DIB – difficulty in breathing. Could be anything. A sixty-four-year-old woman, and the screen tells me she's got COPD, chronic lung disease. Might have nebulisers or home oxygen. Maybe a chest infection that's got out of hand. Likely to be overweight. Hopefully on the ground floor.

I'm there in a few minutes, and find the address but can't get in: there's a wall of hedgerow in front of the house. A voice from the doorstep sends me to the gate round the corner in the next road. The path's overgrown and I have to drag my equipment through the undergrowth. Which means it'll be fun getting the patient out. These are the things that matter.

Thanks for being so quick. It's my mum. She's in the front room.

What's her name?

Mary.

Okay.

I duck through the doorway.

Let's have a chat with Mary.

But Mary is not going to be chatting. She's too busy trying to breathe.

It's an old-fashioned living room. Net curtains in the window, ornaments on the mantel, a floral rug in front of a gas fire. Antimacassars on the three-piece that Mary probably embroidered herself.

Mary is perched on the front edge of the sofa, craning forward as if she's trying to see past someone at a sporting event. But the problem's not her view: she's trying to make her lungs bigger. Her husband clutches a stack of medicines in the chair across from her.

Evening, Mary. You're having trouble with your breathing?

She tries to answer, opens her mouth to explain, but nothing comes out. Instead she purses her lips and blows out air, then immediately sucks it back in.

Can I answer for her?

Her son sits on the arm of the chair.

Absolutely. How long's your mum been unwell?

I take Mary's wrist and feel for a pulse. I'm watching her chest heave up and down, noting the effort and the speed.

I've never seen her this bad. I mean, she's had CPOD for years. Is that right?

COPD, yeah.

Sorry, COPD. But she's never been like this.

How long's it been this bad?

I'm attaching a probe to read her oxygen levels and a blood pressure cuff.

She's been struggling for a while. What do you think, Dad? Three or four days?

The husband nods.

You know. Bit of a cough. Can't get comfortable. Dry throat. This heat . . . But it's only since this afternoon that she's been like this.

I'm going to give her a nebuliser. I pull my stethoscope from my pocket for a quick listen – front, back, under the arms – but all I can hear is the effort – not so much a wheeze, more a general strain of congealed exertion. Her oxygen levels are dropping.

I take a mask from my bag, find the two drugs and squeeze the liquids into the chamber, connect the tubing, switch the dial to eight litres. As I do so I'm firing questions at the son –

Does she have home oxygen? Nebulisers? Any chest pain at all?

– and the son, picking up on the urgency, gives me the concise responses I need:

No. Yes. She hasn't said.

Has she been coughing anything up? What colour?

Yes, just white, I think.

Any fevers? Antibiotics?

A urine infection last month. Otherwise, no.

Has she been sleeping?

She's hardly slept at all in this heat.

Here you go, Mary. Does she lie down or sit up to sleep?

I put the mask over her face.

Last night she couldn't get up the stairs.

Some medicine for your breathing. And that's unusual?

Yes.

Are her ankles swollen? Take some deep breaths, Mary.

She ended up sleeping in the armchair.

Has she been walking about?

Hardly. She's getting more and more exhausted.

As if to endorse her son's words, right in front of my eyes Mary is running out of steam. The labour of each breath is too much for its reward, and I can see her body discarding all other concerns to focus on this one task. When I arrived she'd held my gaze, but now her eyes have a faraway, inward look. Her upright posture has subsided to a wearied slouch. Her skin has taken on a pallid sheen.

Mary? Can you hear me, Mary?

And then it happens. Her final breath.

No great gasp. No tumble to the floor. She simply takes a breath – and then fails to take another.

I've been in the house less than three minutes.

★

The moment the light goes out is always a shock. The final exhalation and the absence that follows. The loss of power as if a lead has been pulled. The corporeal slump of capitulation. It's a gut-punch. Even when I can see it coming, it always arrives too soon. Of course it does.

Ambulances often arrive after the fact – when the terminal blackout has already occurred. Crews find a patient in cardiac arrest and slip into resuscitation mode. They know where they are with cardiac arrests: page one of the ambulance manual, a well-practised drill. Patients in arrest have no personality, no past. To be brutal, for the patient who's stopped breathing, things can't get any worse.

The patient in rapid decline presents a different challenge. This is the moment of opportunity. The tiny arena of intervention. Time is of the essence. Beneath the surface irreparable damage is occurring. All the signs point to a fatal outcome. But the crew attempts to reverse the plunge.

And then the threat is realised: the body succumbs. Expected, inevitable, it's still a moment of failure, a pang of cruelty unremarked in the seamless shift of momentum. For this patient, a moment ago caught in a downward spiral, things have suddenly got as bad as they can get.

I grab the patient's shoulder and shake.

Mary?

I feel the crook of the neck for a pulse. The son watches my every move.

What's happened?

I need to get the patient flat.

What's going on?

There's no time for niceties.

Your mum's stopped breathing, can you help me get her on the floor?

This is a monstrous sentence to utter, and an even tougher one to hear. But there's no pause from the son. He doesn't buckle, or freeze, or bury his face in his hands. He will save his distress for the private future; in this moment he'll be the world's pragmatic deputy, because right now that's what his mum needs and there's no one else to step in. The husband is frozen on the sofa, gripping the medicine boxes on his lap.

The son takes hold of a shoulder and we spin the patient and lower her to the carpet, and I pull her into the space in the middle of her living-room floor. I kneel behind her head, looking down the length of her body, pull the bag and the defib towards me, drag her blouse indecorously up to her armpits, exposing the unlit flesh of her torso, slap on the pads, grab the bag-valve mask, plug it into the oxygen, hold the mask over her face, squeeze in a breath, then another, then another, then another, watching the screen for the heart trace to register. It shows up as a valid rhythm – what you might see if Mary was still talking. I feel her neck again – nothing. I move my hand – are my fingers in the wrong place? This is the omnipresent doubt – that, after all this time, I could still bungle something as basic as feeling a pulse. Is it just incredibly faint? Too much flesh in the way? Still a blank. With the thumb and forefinger of my left hand I clamp the mask in place, squeezing the bag with the right; the second finger pulls the chin towards it; the other two move around the groove in the neck in search of the reassuring throb of circulation. But it's a false hope: there is none.

I drop the BVM and press *priority* on my radio. I lock my hands and lean forward and start pushing on the patient's chest. *One, two, three, four*, pushing down as hard as I can, *five, six, seven, eight* . . . Almost immediately, a cascade of gastric contents erupts from the patient's mouth. A volatile purée of lurid juices, it discharges upwards and spills and sprays and splatters over her face, around her mouth, onto her chin and neck, in lumps across her cheeks and forehead, sliding down into the hollows of her eyes. With each compression of the chest, it gushes indiscriminately outwards, onto her hair and clothing and my outstretched forearms and gloves, and in nonchalant orange splashes across the immaculate floral rug. It's as horrific as it sounds, but there's no time to comment.

I stop my compressions and scoop my arms around her head and under her shoulders and tilt her forcefully onto her left side, pushing my knee behind her back to hold her in place for a few seconds as the rancid concoction pours from her mouth and slides from her skin and falls in a garish, macerated puddle on the rug. It's ghastly and wretched, a biological insult, as if someone is using a luminous highlighter to emphasise the words, SOMETHING REALLY BAD IS HAPPENING HERE. I glance up to see Mary's husband and son looking on in horror.

I'm so sorry about this.

You do what you need to do. Is there anything we can do?

Some tissue or kitchen roll?

My radio beeps. I pull it off my belt clip with a slimy

gloved hand: I should remove the glove but in this clammy heat I'll never get another one back on.

Patient now in cardiac arrest. Can you please dispatch a crew?

We'll have someone with you as soon as we can.

It's handover time, when the day shifts are finishing and the nights are about to start. There's never a good time to suffer a cardiac arrest, but this is one of the worst. I'm going to be on my own for a while.

I rummage around for the hand-held suction. The patient's still on her side, but I want to get her flat again and carry on with the compressions. The son holds out a box of tissues, and I crudely smear the gastric contents away from the patient's mouth, her nose, her eyes. The flow seems to have subsided but I'm sure it will resume when I get back on her chest. I lower her again and open the mouth and insert the nozzle of the suction, squeeze the bulb and release, and the bilious juices are drawn up the tube, but so are several solid chunks, which get stuck in the tubing, and when I squeeze again, the pressure's reduced and nothing more comes out. I clear what I can, but this simple tool is not going to be much help if there's another surge.

I squeeze a few ventilations and go back to the chest, begin the rhythmic impulses. But what I have now is a dilemma.

It's true that working on the car had kept my anxieties gainfully employed, because there was a whole new array of pitfalls to worry about. But there was also a kind of liberation to working alone. Being unable to go anywhere, I found, tended to focus the mind. You could hardly stand around, grinning inanely and saying things like:

I'm sure my colleagues'll be here soon.

You had to *do* something. You had to *act*.

I stripped things down to the essentials. The first two minutes were key. I concerned myself with one task: identifying if a situation was life-threatening (or time-critical). This was my main purpose, and everything else followed from it – or fell away. If it were, I would give as much treatment, take as much history, get things as advanced as possible, in the window before the crew arrived, however long that turned out to be. (And sometimes it was a very long time.)

Rather than feeling inhibited by being alone, I found the responsibility was its own release. It wasn't so much that I could assess patients without being watched and give treatment under my own facility, it was rather that I had to – because there was no one else to do it for me. Against my expectations, I found myself operating with a surprisingly clear mind.

However, there were still moments, as with Mary today, when I needed to do two things – both of them essential – at the same time, with only one pair of hands.

A multitude of factors affect the chances of survival from cardiac arrest, but there are three things that significantly improve patient outcomes:

- *delivering an early shock to a quivering heart*
- *giving effective, continuous chest compressions to maintain circulation*
- *treating any reversible cause of the arrest.*

In Mary's case, the first of these is irrelevant: her heart is in a normal electrical rhythm (at least, for the moment), just not beating properly. But the second and third elements are currently in conflict with each other, and as long as I'm on my own, I can't address them both at once.

As a lone responder, my top priority is providing good-quality CPR – the rhythmical pummelling of the chest to imitate the pumping action of the heart and send blood round the body to the tissues and organs. But I'm confident I'm working with a hypoxic arrest – the patient's breathing problems are the cause – and I need to reoxygenate her so that the blood has a cargo. The problem is that discharge from her stomach: it's soiling the airway, invading the lungs, scorching the tissues, reducing the delivery of oxygen, undermining everything I do.

The treatment is suction, but my equipment has failed. I have a more powerful, electronic machine in the boot of the car, but to fetch it would take about a minute – a small lifetime right now. It's the old quandary: should I stay or should I go? My instincts rebel at the thought of leaving: you don't interrupt CPR for anything; you might as well give up. Conversely, what's the point of pumping away at the circulation if there's no oxygen getting in because the airway's filled with vomit?

My reluctance to abandon a critically ill patient wins out: I stay and continue basic life support, clearing the airway as best I can with my improvised tools and some repositioning, and trusting back-up will soon arrive. Her chest is moving when I squeeze the bag, so there's some air going in. After what feels like many minutes, a crew does show up, and suddenly there are more hands – to take over CPR, to fetch what we need, to suction the debris from the mouth and throat, to place an advanced airway device which will protect the lungs from more regurgitated poison, to pierce the vein and administer the relevant resuscitation drugs.

We take on our various roles and, apart from some logistical hitches, work as the well-rehearsed crew from the training script. The son and husband watch, shell-shocked, as the reality begins to sink in. After a short while the target moment occurs and we can feel a pulse: Mary's heart is beating for itself. But there's none of that sense of elation this time.

Any ROSC (return of spontaneous circulation) is a significant moment, of course, but at this stage hope still hangs in the balance. I suspect the adrenaline is working its magic, increasing the power of the heart's contractions, but the question is whether the body can sustain its circulation once we take our hands away and leave it to its own devices.

For a few minutes it does so, but then the blood pressure drops and the pulse fades and in spite of some supportive treatment, the patient goes back into arrest. The process is repeated a couple of times: we push, squeeze, medicate; we identify a pulse again, but the moment is short-lived and we resuscitate again.

Caught in a repeating cycle, we decide to move to hospital. We package the patient and carry her out through the undergrowth to the ambulance. We set off to hospital with a pre-alert of what's coming in. When we arrive, I give a verbal handover to the waiting team, and they take charge. And suddenly, like that, our work is done. We watch for a few minutes, then head outside.

In the days that follow Mary's collapse, I worry I did the wrong thing. These are the standard misgivings. On what basis did I choose my course? Did I consider all the options in the heat of the moment? Was my thinking affected by being on my own? Was my decision made with a clear mind backed by sound rationale, weighing the potential impacts? Or, in the tension of the situation, was I acting with a kind of panicked intuition?

I realise in hindsight I could have sent the son out to the car for the more powerful suction unit. At the time the thought had crossed my mind, but been rejected because of the difficulty of removing the machine from its mount – a complicated process to explain, one I had struggled with myself as a newcomer. Could I have asked him to perform chest compressions while I fetched it myself? This would have been traumatic for him, and it's unlikely the compressions would have been effective, but it would have been better than nothing. In the post-match analysis, there are several alternatives, and compelling arguments on each side.

I ask my peers and superiors what they would have done – unsure if I'm looking for endorsement or criticism. No one has a definitive answer, which I suppose is reassuring, and it seems unlikely a different course would have changed the outcome. But that doesn't mean there's nothing to learn; nor does it silence the internal debate.

What I'm processing is the reality that there's a downside

to all this. That being the rescuer won't always work out, and you can't avoid the spectre of failure – and being responsible for that failure – for ever. To intervene in someone's situation is a privilege, of course, and especially in an emergency. But the consequences are not always positive, and the more ill someone is, the higher the stakes become. The truth is that any situation that's worth trying to fix can just as easily be made worse.

Although I could have tried something different for Mary, on reflection, I think I did everything I could. Yet the mistake with serious, maybe disastrous, consequences is always waiting just around the corner. There are only two ways to avoid this: the first is to be perfect; the second is never to go to anyone really ill (or find some other way to make a living). Option one may be impossible, but as an aspiration, it's preferable to its alternative.

We are completing our paperwork in the ambulance at hospital. Cleaning, restocking, refreshing; offloading our casual morbidity with biscuits and dark humour before we move on to the next call of the airless night.

The patient's son and husband approach the back of the ambulance.

Hello? Sorry to interrupt.

I step down from the truck. I'm warm, sweaty, clutching a bottle of water. They stand close together. It's the son who speaks.

We just wanted to thank you for what you did. We saw how hard you worked.

Not at all. I'm sorry it was so traumatic. So . . . unpleasant.

The husband's eyes are red, but dry. The inference is clear: the hospital have stopped resuscitating, and Mary has died. But I don't know this for sure – we've been outside since handing over – so I'm careful with my words. I can't offer condolences in case I'm wrong. But the interaction needs a phrase of closure.

It's very kind of you to come and speak to me . . . at a time like this.
We wanted you to know how grateful we are.

The son shakes my hand.

Thank you.

They turn and walk back into the hospital. The son rests his hand on his father's shoulder.

XV

Sharon is still on the phone when she opens her front door and spots the police.

Oh!

It's the first haze of dawn. She extends a finger and counts the uniforms in turn.

I didn't call the police. Where's the ambulance?

The first officer nods in my direction: I give a little wave. She returns to her call, her voice now pierced with a hint of pique.

Sorry, darling. I've got three burly policemen on my doorstep? And a skinny paramedic? I didn't ask for police.

The officer steps forward.

We're only here because of what you said.

What was that then?

You told them you were holding a knife to your throat.

You're not coming in my house.

It's up to you. But the paramedic can't come in without us.

She stares hard, listening or thinking.

You can come in. The other two can wait outside.

What about that knife, Sharon?

Oh, you know my name already? And you haven't even bought me a drink yet! You're very forward, Mr Policeman . . .

She leans against the doorway and crosses one leg over the other. A thigh emerges from her scarlet robe.

Wait, have we met before? Let me see your left hand. No wedding ring!

Where's the knife, Sharon?

In the kitchen. With the forks and spoons. Where do you keep your cutlery?

You know how this works, Sharon. We're here for your welfare.

Do you want to search me?

She pulls at the lapels of her robe, flicking it half-open and closed again, then stops, glares at the officer, holding his gaze. Then breaks into a throaty cackle.

I'm only playing with you. Oh! So serious! What's wrong, babe? Long night?

She holds out her hand and smacks herself on the wrist –

Trying to be too friendly. That's always been my problem. Too much to say for myself.

– then disappears down the hallway, still talking, confident we'll follow.

The house is a diorama of her restless mind. Ethnic drapes and moody lamps give the drowsy feel of a boudoir, but there's an angry scorch mark on the rug and an empty bottle of Archer's on the floor. A black and white cat darts out of the kitchen and scurries behind a sofa strewn with crumpled clothes and heart-shaped cushions stitched with 'LUV U 4

EVER' and 'World's Best Mum'. The mantel is decorated with scented candles and joss sticks, soft toys and birthday cards. On the walls, photos of children in school uniform are interspersed with studio shots of a lingerie-clad woman – is that Sharon in her younger years?

That's what I've always been told. Don't know when to stop. Too damn mouthy by half. That's why I don't get no help. They don't know how to handle me. What, just because I say it how it is? Just because I can see through their bullshit? Just because I'm not Little Miss Sunshine, Skinny Hippy Vegan Goody Two Shoes? I mean, what do they expect? I can't help it. That's what they're for, isn't it? Isn't it?

She looks at me.

Well? Isn't it? Are you going to join in, or just leave me talking to myself here?

Sharon . . .

He speaks! For a moment I thought you were just going to stare! Don't be shy, babe.

Can you tell me what's happened tonight?

Uuuhhhh! Can't you guys think of something more original to ask? That's what they all say. Not much of a chat-up line, is it?

I guess not.

Do you want to give it another go?

Not really, Sharon.

Oh, I see. We've got a grumpy one tonight.

I'd just like to know what's wrong, Sharon. So we can help you.

Well that depends. Aren't you going to introduce yourself?

She puts out her hand, folded at the wrist. A princess waiting to be anointed with a kiss – or a Labrador expecting a treat. I give the hand a brisk, business-like shake.

Jake.

Are you married, Jake?

I laugh, once, as if she's made a joke.

Well?

Can you tell me why you called the ambulance?

Ah-ah-ahhh! Don't avoid my question . . .!

She lights a couple of tea-lights, tossing the match unseen onto the rug; the flame disappears as it falls, but I keep glancing down just to make sure.

I'm not avoiding your question, Sharon.

So what's the answer, handsome?

I just don't think it's relevant.

I can see the ring through your glove!

She places the tea-lights inside ceramic burners and adds some oil, inhaling luxuriantly.

You see how smart I am? I could be your boss.

I'm sure you could.

You lot are all the same. You come in here with that look on your face. Can't wait to leave, can you? Can't wait to get away.

That's not the case.

You think I'm stupid.

Sharon, I'm just trying to concentrate on the matter at hand.

Which is?

Why don't you tell me what's happened? You still haven't told me why you called.

I'll tell you what, Jake. Is that really your name? I'll tell you why I called if you smile at me. You're a pretty little thing, aren't you? Like a little choirboy. But so serious. Just a smile. Will you give me a smile, Jake? Just a little smile?

Sharon . . .

Even half a smile? Just the left-hand side of your face?

She pokes her cheek with her index finger, forcing her mouth into an emotionless curl.

You see? It's not difficult.

Perhaps on another day, another night, I would have the energy to smile. To indulge Sharon, to oil the cogs, maybe even tease her a little, but not too much; to scratch whatever itch has provoked her call.

As time rolls on – and on, and on – Sharon becomes increasingly belligerent. She talks vaguely about self-harm, makes opaque references to previous injustices and her chaotic home life. Cancelled meetings with social workers, hostile encounters with support workers, angry answerphone messages left at three a.m. A hundred reasons why everyone's got the wrong idea. But she won't answer a direct question, won't tell me why we're here, and every suggestion I make is met with a snub: she refuses hospital, insists there's no one we can call, ridicules any attempt to refer her to a psychiatric team, claiming she's had contact with all the available resources and none of them can handle her.

Sharon, do you have any medical conditions?

You know I do.

What are they?

Mental health, mental health. It's all fucking mental health.

Which mental health?

She squints disdainfully, slams her hand down on the arm of the chair.

I have a chemical imbalance in my brain, okay? I'm not making this up. I'm not trying to get attention.

She stands and starts pacing.

I'm certainly not suggesting that, Sharon. Have you been diagnosed with a particular psychiatric condition?

Hah! Like you don't already know! Everyone knows me. Everyone knows Sharon Smith.

Now she reaches her arm down behind the sofa. The officer steps forward, which seems to amuse her –

Don't worry, Mr Policeman!

– as she lifts the cat from its hiding place, swooping it up in a dramatic arc, as if she's going to throw it, then depositing it in the crook of her arm, nuzzling the top of its head and massaging the backs of its ears.

You got children, Jake?

I'm sorry?

Have you got children?

Sharon, you didn't call an ambulance to ask me about my kids, did you?

Didn't I? How do you know?

Why don't you tell me what the problem is?

What are their names?

The cat purrs loudly.

Sharon, we're not getting very far, are we?

Are you frightened to tell me? What do you think I'm going to do? Come to your house and kidnap them? Abuse them? Steal your fucking kids from you? Like they did to me?

She tips the cat onto the floor and points at my forehead. Anger floods her face.

Can you imagine that? Someone taking your kids? Because of something someone else has done? Because of something someone did to them. And I'm the one left here on my own. On my fucking birthday. Drinking peach schnapps and holding a knife to my throat. Again. Yeah! That's right! Again! Always threatening! And calling for help and having the police turn up on my doorstep where everyone can see them. Oh, Sharon's got the police round again! What's she done this time? Driven her car into the front wall? Smashed up her flat? Set her curtains on fire? You wanna know what my diagnosis is? Here!

She grabs a box of medication and throws it across the room. I catch the box and look at the name just as a second box –

Here!

– flies past my head. And a third.

Here!

Box after box, she throws her medicines across the room at me.

Here! Here! Here! Here! Here! Here!

It goes on and on. Back and forth. It's as if we're trapped in an airport lounge – where the departure boards have glitched and the letters keep rotating endlessly through the alphabet. Some of the long-term problems are clear. But as for today's specific issue, and what we can do about it, I'm still none the wiser after more than two hours. Sharon won't leave the house; nor will she let us call anyone on her behalf. Yet when I or the police talk about leaving, she grabs a knife and waves it around, or switches on the gas in the kitchen. I don't think it's unfair to say that she does these things wilfully, even inventively. She is, to be frank, a skilled, perhaps even devious negotiator. But if she's negotiating, what I can't figure out is what she's negotiating towards. What is her ultimate goal? What does she *want*? There's something prosaic about her actions, as if she's going through the motions, but that doesn't mean she's not willing to go through with it – as I'm soon to find out.

I know you don't like the questions, Sharon, but we can't help if we don't know what you want.

She is sat cross-legged on the sofa now, tapping at her phone – the phone she has already told me is out of battery.

We're left with, I think, two options.

I'm not going to A&E. I'm not going anywhere.

Tap, tap, tap.

Okay. So I could refer you to –

The crisis team? That's what you're going to say. You see? I know all your tactics. I'm a fucking veteran. And the answer's no.

Why not? Sharon . . .? What do you want?

Anyone ever told you you've got the face of a headmaster? Talking to you's like being back at school. No sense of humour. Maybe you're in the wrong job, have you thought about a change of career? Godddd! I'm trying to tell you about the crap going on in my life. And you keep saying the same thing, over and over, 'Why did you call? Why did you call? Why did you call?' You're like a parrot!

Sharon . . .

Stop saying my name like that!

I wait.

You bastards are all the same. Ambulance. Police. Crisis team. You make out you care, ask me all these questions in your soft little reassuring fucking patronising voices. But you don't give a shit. You can't wait to leave, can you? I'm just a fucking inconvenience to you. You're just trying to find a way to palm me off on someone else. 'Let us take you to A&E, Sharon. Let us refer you to the crisis team.' Yeah, so you can go off and do something more interesting. Drive to the garage and get your free coffee. Look after someone who's not such a giant pain in the arse!

She may be right about the availability of care, but there's an obstructive egotism to this claim that she's somehow exceptional and therefore out of reach. I wonder if she knows how many times I've heard it before. She's not the first one to claim she's impossible to help, then behave impossibly to prove herself right.

In truth, I think what she wants is company. For all the bluster, the coquettishness, the antagonism; for all the claims that she's too special to be helped, too hostile for affection, too broken for repair, that she's beyond the communal hand-hold, Sharon is in the end, I suspect, a lonely human being who wants someone to spend some time with her – albeit one who uses attack and destruction to get attention, who brandishes weapons at those she's called for help, who throws herself on the floor and expects to be lifted up, who wakes her neighbours at two a.m. by tipping her furniture out of the first-floor window. Perhaps the central tragedy of all this is that she's unable to apply her ingenuity to an alternative – not to the manipulation of elaborate scenarios such as the one I now find myself in, but to the kind of relationships that might fulfil the needs for which she is currently, on an almost daily basis, drafting in the emergency services.

Sharon, do you really think that? Do you really think that, as a profession, as individuals, we actively try not to help you?

Babe, I can see it in your eyes. You don't wanna be here. You don't wanna help me. You're just like all the others. Your mates who came here last time. The nurses in A&E who look at me like I'm shit. The crisis team with their massive arses: 'Sohh, Shar-rohnn . . . What iz de problem? Let me sit my fat arse dowwwn and we can talllk about eet.' They can't deal with me. I'm too much trouble.

She gives me a slow, hateful stare –

Too. Fucking. Complicated.

– and walks out of the room.

I have to offer her something. She's called out for help. Everything she's done since I've got here has confused and hampered that process, but the principle remains. Hospital is not an option. The best I can do is to refer her to the massive-arsed crisis team. So I make the call. Amazingly, someone answers the phone. They can't speak to her now, they say, but they agree to call Sharon in the morning, in office hours, with a view to coming to see her. I head up the stairs to the landing to break the news. Sharon's leaning over the balustrade, smoking a cigarette under the supervision of the police officer.

Sharon. I take it you haven't changed your mind about hospital?

Has the hospital changed its mind about me?

So I've called the crisis team for you.

Dumping me on some other poor bastard?

Someone's going to call you in the morning. Well, later today, in fact. In about five hours.

I'll be asleep.

Try not to be.

Hah!

They'll have a chat with you over the phone. And then they might come round and see you.

I told you already I'm not interested.

Okay but you've called asking for help.

Not that kind of help.

And I'm trying to find you some help. It may not be perfect, Sharon. But I don't want to leave you with nothing.

You mean you don't want to get in trouble.

No.

She flicks her cigarette away in an arc without looking. It drops onto the floor below.

Sharon?

She ducks into the bedroom and goes to shut the door, but the officer extends an arm and pushes it back open. It's a flimsy piece of board with boulder-dents at knee and shoulder height. She hooks her hands onto it and tries to swing it shut, but his arm stands firm.

Oh, is that how's it going to be?

Sharon . . .

She pushes past him out of the room and marches round the landing to the top of the stairs. Before we're able to say or do anything, she leans forward – and tips herself down the stairs. It's not a fall and it's not a jump – she just leans forward and goes. No histrionics, no warning. As simple as that. There's no time to react.

Sharon!

She plummets downwards, rolling, tumbling, rattling down

the thinly carpeted stairs. It's at once both shocking and utterly casual. Her body slides and spins, and then clatters into the wall at the bottom of the stairs and topples sideways. She comes to rest in the middle of the hallway, her robe barely covering her, a bundle of exposed and motionless flesh. It's all over in a couple of seconds.

I think I swear under my breath.

Sharon? Sharon?

I skip down the steps two at a time, and crouch down at her shoulder. Instinctively, my boot stretches to the cigarette butt and crushes it, just in case. I give Sharon a pain stimulus on her trapezius, but there's no reaction. I feel her wrist to confirm a pulse, put an oxygen mask on her face, shine a light in her eyes, then run my hands over her head, checking for lumps or bleeding or worse. Then I press in on my radio to ask for a truck. This is a new scenario and there'll be no debate about hospital now. I perform some of the basic checks she wouldn't allow in her earlier state – heart rate, blood pressure and so on. I tie a tourniquet round her arm for a cannula. She flinches and begins to stir.

Are you awake, Sharon? Can you hear me? It's the ambulance. Can you open your eyes, Sharon?

Her eyes don't open, but there's a wince at the eyebrows, a flicker of movement along the lashes.

It's going to be okay, Sharon. Do you know where you are? You're in your house.

The eyelids wobble.

It's the ambulance. You fell down the stairs.

And now her eyes open, and she looks straight at me.

167

Sharon. Try to keep still.
Her stare is unblinking.
We're going to take you to hospital.
No you're not.
I'm relieved to hear her speak.
Tell me where it hurts.
I'm not going anywhere.

XVI

The junction's not quite a crossroads; it's more like a pair of forks in the road, one impaled on the other, the tines twisted off to the sides. Multiple lanes span the wide expanse of tarmac, with the feel of an airport runway and the destination options daubed in shorthand on the ground.

Street lamps drop their pools of enlightenment like stooping giants, and traffic lights pierce the night sky in all directions, endlessly instructing. Engines growl their impatience and horns squawk their discontent. Pedestrians hover on the fenced-off islands; cyclists slalom through to reach their boxes at the front. When the lights change, the cars and vans will throttle away and undertake each other, and the mopeds will swerve into oncoming traffic with their apologetic L plates, because they can't afford to be late.

This is an intersection in the true sense of the word, a meeting of worlds, a place for hopping off and hopping on. Cafés, minimarkets and street vendors sell their wares; the voluntary and the employed hand out leaflets, menus, newspapers and tracts. Most glide by on the way to somewhere else, but many linger: at coffee tables, on benches; those with nowhere else to go. One man shouts from knee-height at passers-by, another holds a sign of general condemnation; a third does pull-ups in Lycra on one of the road signs.

There's a sense of urgency in the air, and it comes from the road and the station and the pace of city life. Buried in timetables and congestion, expressed in the grammar of an urban blues. Friction, combustion, alarms, promises; music, motion, sirens, rage. Forever stopping and starting and stopping again.

The left lanes belong to the buses, swooping in to hoover up their consignments before lurching back out, jostling to maintain their position in the onward flow. One of them pulls up heading east, and already the passengers, peering through the steamed-up windows, have spotted their connection across the road, heading south, three crossings away. They spill off and scurry to the lights, shopping bags and toddlers trailing behind, but the sequence is against them, and they're only at the island when their double-decker carriage pulls away; the only people who've made it are the ones who skipped the lights and made a reckless dash across the six lanes. One of them has only got halfway when the lights change again, and he's stranded, embarrassed, looking this way and that, until the lights change and he can scamper to the opposite shore, laughing with a couple of strangers who have spotted his plight.

These negotiations go on through the day and most of the night; a congregation of nobodies making their way in the world, saving a few minutes, trying to get home. And this is how it happens. Aware of the dangers, informed of the risks, able to read the yellow incident signs along the kerb. Confident that probability will protect them, and that tragedy will find its quarry somewhere else.

The patient's in the road, his head on the kerb like a pillow. It's dark and he's in the shadow of the bus, right next to a bin. His face and hair are caked with blood. His jacket's ripped, his clothing scuffed with dirt, his legs skewed awkwardly to the left. One of his shoes has come off.

The job's come down as a cardiac arrest, but I can see he's breathing. There's a responder on scene, another FRU, who came across this as a running call. There are people and vehicles all around: bustle, haste, clamour, glare. It's ten o'clock at night.

We're a short way past the stop, and the bus has its hazards on to block the lane. I pull up beside it to give us some more protection, but the traffic keeps squeezing through, pausing for a glimpse, then racing away.

Before I've even reached the patient, my radio buzzes and I'm asked for a report. I tell the controller what I can see: the patient's injured but not dead, more details to follow, and they tell me the trauma team has been dispatched. I touch the responder's shoulder.

Hello, mate. What do you need?

Just trying to work out his injuries. So he's about forty, I think. Hit by a car.

Anyone see what happened?

He stepped out from behind the bus by the sound of it.

We're twenty yards from a pedestrian crossing.

Driver says he was doing thirty – who knows? Bull's-eyed the windscreen apparently. Haven't seen the damage myself. Car's down there.

I glance down the road. It's a thoroughbred saloon with blacked-out windows about a hundred yards away – a long way past if you've hit someone doing thirty.

Okay. The trauma team's on the way.

I move round behind the patient and place my hands on his shoulders.

It's the ambulance, my friend. Can you hear me? We need you to keep still. Try not to move.

I move my hands up to the sides of his head. My colleague's been preparing oxygen, and now he reaches out the mask to hook it onto the patient's face – but the patient squirms and groans and pushes it away. This is not what we want. He's had a high-mechanism impact and we have to suspect a spinal fracture. We want to keep him still. Any unnecessary movement could cause catastrophic nerve damage.

We're going to help you. Try to stay still.

I try to hold him, but this just upsets him – he flails his arm to push me away and half sits up and turns his head. He tries to shout something but it's a muffled growl, trapped in his throat or his sluggish brain. I'm not sure if the sounds he's making are words or noises – the fruit of a concussion, a drunken grievance? We're going to struggle to reason with him.

The crowd at the bus stop watches the saga unfolding a few yards from their feet. No one makes suggestions or tries to interfere – which is surprising. Normally there'd be a local expert or two, someone offering a commentary or talking about compensation, but I think they can sense that tonight they should leave it to the people with the blue lights.

When it comes to trauma, ambulance crews like to play it cool. Appearances are vital, so it's important to make out you've seen it all before. Mangled extremities and amputations? Old news. Fatal car crashes? Yeah, whatever. Multiple stabbings? All in a day's work . . .

The truth is not so simple. You'd never get anyone to admit it, but most people in the job are just as fascinated by the gory and gruesome calls as your average *Casualty* viewer – they just get their buzz from the real world instead of a rectangular screen in the corner of the living room. Shootings, bodies on the tracks, falls from height: these are the glamour jobs of the emergency world. They're the stuff of good drama because they're life-changing moments that have come out of nowhere, and life and death still hang in the balance. The reverence accorded to these jobs is just as prevalent in the mess rooms of ambulance stations across the country as it is in the wider public – it just takes a more sardonic, nonchalant form.

So, if you have a lively shift, your crewmate might utter the notorious phrase:

I'm never working with you again!

Go to a run of nasty jobs and your colleagues might start calling you Dr Death or Trauma Magnet. These are jocular accusations that you're somehow working too close to the flame, but they're also an acknowledgement that you've earned your stripes in the world of emergency care.

No one ever asks you about the three hours you spent with a suicidal psychiatric patient, persuading them to come to hospital because their capacity was in doubt and you knew they needed help and support. But turn up first to a car that's been wrapped around a tree, and where there's nothing to do because the patient's injuries are incompatible with life, and everyone will be asking you the grisly details for the next fortnight.

In the early days, I'd fallen for this myth. If I wasn't saving a life or a limb on a daily basis, I thought that meant I was somehow deficient – as if a higher power were controlling which vehicles went where, and didn't trust me with one of the jobs on the venerated list. I taunted myself with the calls I was yet to cross off (mainly of a traumatic nature), and resented the implicit failings of which they spoke:

Been to a fatal stabbing yet? No? Not seen them open up the chest? What about a nasty RTC? A traumatic arrest? You don't do a lot of trauma, do you? What, you haven't been to a shooting yet? Even working round here?

Of course, it was nonsense. Such value judgements about the status of different jobs are insultingly crude. They come from the same place that determines that young men who've been stabbed in the leg get a multi-resource response within a few minutes, while elderly patients with a fractured hip have to wait several hours for any kind of help. To us, these major traumas and casual fatalities were mere ornaments of our working lives. But for each one we notched up, there was a real impact somewhere – a loss, a brokenness, a

174

devastation – even if they were suffered by someone we'd never have to look in the eye.

The patient's face is a gallery of bruises and scars, only some from today. His nose has veered sideways, no longer perpendicular to his face. He's far from fully alert. Whatever we do to settle him down seems to have the opposite effect, so my colleague's abandoned the oxygen and is checking his chest, his head, his neck, his limbs, lifting clothes, feeling with his palms, gently pressing but trying not to upset him in the process. On the scale we use to assess consciousness, I'd give the patient about nine out of fifteen: he's groaning, trying to speak; his eyes are closed. I don't think he knows what's going on.

I've let go of his head and he's stopped trying to move away, but we can't stay hands-off for ever. We need to find the physical outcomes of his encounter with high-speed metal. We're not going to fix him here, but we need to protect him from further damage and halt any deterioration; we need to package him and move him and make him comfortable if we can. We might need to make some more critical interventions. And all as quickly as we can. None of this seems feasible right now.

Another ambulance car arrives – it's going to be one of those jobs where everyone turns up, because it's been given as a cardiac arrest and it's in a very public place. This one has a responder and a student on board, keen to get stuck into something fruity. The police are here too, and they set about closing the road, sending the relentless traffic down another route. But no transporting ambulance yet.

We start cutting off clothes, exposing flesh to look for

damage, up the limbs and towards the torso, covering with a blanket, trying to maintain some dignity in the middle of this circus. There are friction burns along his arm and his chest: as if he's sustained road rash through his clothes. We try to feel his ribs, but this just makes him flinch. There's what looks like bruising, probably some deeper injuries too.

Someone's checked the car for damage:

There's a big dent in the bonnet, one of the lights is smashed. And the windscreen. It's not just bull's-eyed. It's completely caved in on the passenger side. It's a hell of an impact. I'd be amazed if that happened at thirty.

The guy who was here first is trying to get some obs. He's put a little probe on the patient's finger and he's trying to attach a blood pressure cuff. But the patient's having none of it; he's becoming more and more combative, pushing away, trying to stand up, unable to fathom why all these people are harassing him.

We've managed to find his wallet so we have a name: Pawel. He has no companion with him, no family or friend to assist us, to reassure him, to fill in the blanks. Where is he from? To whom does he belong?

Pawel, Pawel. Try and stay calm.

Where are the people who know him and care about him? Are they in another country? Wherever they are, they don't know yet what's happened to him.

Pawel, my friend. We're trying to help you.

I doubt he can understand; I don't even know if he can hear me. I try to reassure him with the tone of my voice. But it's lost in the twilight commotion of everything going on.

A fourth ambulance car arrives, and there's someone else to explain the situation to, someone else to throw their views into the mix. The patient now has five people around him but it feels like nothing's getting done. You know the phrase about too many cooks . . .

Can we get some O$_2$ on him?

We've tried that –

And we need to immobilise.

If only we could, mate . . .

He won't let us touch him.

He's very combative.

Have we asked for the trauma team?

They're on the way.

I'm worried things are drifting – or going round on a loop. I sense that I should be more assertive, but I wasn't here first and something holds me back. I'm away from my normal area and I don't know the others on scene. Am I relying on the doctor to turn up and take command? Or am I wary of sounding like a hotshot, afraid that if I grab the reins the next thing I'll do is fall on my backside?

Maybe I'm waiting for that more heroic version of myself to turn up – the one I always imagined would materialise on such occasions. The one who stands with his feet wide apart and his shoulders back, who lifts his chin and looks people in the eye with cool authority, who speaks an octave lower than everyone else. The one the rain bounces off; the one who never feels the cold.

People joke about ambulance crews putting on their super-hero outfits – as if those baggy green combats hold mysterious powers to engender calm. Like the vast majority of my colleagues, I've never considered this a heroic job, but I did have a vague expectation that it would bring out something different in me; that certain situations would require a kind of enhanced version of reality, and so a more commanding manifestation would suddenly drop in from somewhere and take control.

The reality is far simpler. The reality is that I'm here and this is normal and I'm getting on with it just the same. I am the same me who's intimidated by bar staff with big beards and who wears two pairs of socks on night shifts in winter, and this doesn't mean I cannot help. I am not transformed. I am a fairly normal person, doing a slightly abnormal thing.

Since we can't control the patient in his current state, I decide to try to get a needle in his arm. At least when the doctor arrives, he or she can give something to relax the patient, or even knock him out. Then the other problems can be addressed.

Can you give me a hand?

The patient's sitting up now, mumbling and starting to open his eyes – if anything, more restless than before. I imagine, if you were injured and sore, and unsure what's happened or where you were, the last thing you'd want would be for a group of strangers to gather round you, and for one of them to try to stab you in the arm – so I proceed with a decent slab of caution.

I wrap a tourniquet around his right arm. My colleague attaches the BP cuff on the other side – I doubt we'll get a reading, but it might distract the patient long enough.

It's okay, mate. We're here to help.

There's a nice prominent vein in the crook of his arm: I take hold of his wrist. The cuff begins inflating and he looks down at his left arm, and I slide the cannula in as smoothly as I can in the right. For a moment he's still, and there's a flashback in the chamber, so I retract the needle and take it away, screwing the cap on just before the patient suddenly feels this latest wound, five seconds too late, and pulls his arm away.

Pawel . . .

Now he's trying to stand. I see the ambulance pulling in. He pulls off the blood pressure cuff, looks all around, seeing or not seeing, completely bewildered, unable to get himself up, and leans back again. The car with the trauma team arrives as well. The cannula is lodged in the vein of his right arm, but not secured. As he waves his arm, the tiny plastic apparatus flaps about, in danger of flying out at any moment. One of my colleagues grabs his arm and holds it still, and we manage to apply some tape, then wind a dressing round and round for good measure.

By the time this little mission is complete, we have another six people with us – three from the trauma team and three from the ambulance. Some days you wait half an hour in the cold and dark before anyone else turns up, trying to explain to the patient and the bystanders why no one else has come to help. Other days a whole football team turns up in green.

My colleague gives a little rundown, and the doctor starts assessing for himself. Maybe he's wondering why we haven't got very far with treatment; maybe he can see the challenges we've had.

Let's make sure we look after that cannula. Is it nice and secure?
Not flushed it yet, but it's taped down and it's definitely in.

Good. I think we'll give something to relax him, then we'll look at an RSI.

Sure enough, within minutes of being given the first medicine, the patient is a new man. We settle him on the trolley bed, and the trauma team set about the rapid sequence intubation – knocking him out and inserting an airway tube. There are many hands on scene to assist, and I step backwards to give them some space. The ambulance crew are the go-to guys now, the custodians, the transporters. As a first responder, I'm suddenly surplus to requirements – a placeholder, a babysitter, a transient. I step away.

Things are suddenly calm. The bus stop has cleared of onlookers. Even the traffic has gone quiet. The patient is loaded onto the ambulance and the back door closes, and just like that, the dazzling public drama disappears into a box. All the tension, all the turmoil has been distilled to one small moment. No swooping rescue or daring intervention. The insertion of a needle into a vein is hardly the stuff of glory, but sometimes it's the simplest of actions that can unlock the door.

XVII

I didn't want an ambulance.

   No?

I told them not to send you.

   Okay.

I said I didn't need you.

   Right.

They said, 'An ambulance will be with you shortly.' 'An ambulance?' I said. 'Why?' 'Don't eat or drink anything, and shut away any pets.' We're not even allowed pets here . . . Then I got worried. I thought, well, maybe there is something wrong? They're the experts, aren't they? But now you're here, well, isn't there someone somewhere who really needs you?

   Don't worry. It happens all the time.

I am a human safety net. A mobile fall guy. A road sweeper. A live-action android, under the command of an algorithm in a distant call-centre. I am a name on a hundred pieces of paperwork all over the city. A hook to hang the blame on.

   It's a crazy night, and they're short of crews. They keep

broadcasting the jobs they're holding, some of them hours old. I'm on a car, so I should be kept for the most serious calls, but whenever I go green, I'm sent to another patient like Andrew.

I'm giving no treatment, confronting no disasters. Not intervening, not rescuing, not alleviating, not changing anything. I'm getting no ambulance to back me up until I ask for it. I'm sure there are sick people somewhere in the city; I just haven't come across one in a very long time. And I'm starting to forget what they look like.

My main purpose on a night like this is to involve as few transporting ambulances as I can in the onward referral of as many patients as possible – as long as it's safe to do so. To smooth out the bumps in a system running on cobbles. And to take responsibility if the unexpected occurs. It's an exercise, primarily, in the exclusion of risk.

Andrew lives with his girlfriend in a block of new-builds that's yet to make it onto the satnav. The door opens into a living area which incorporates the kitchen with the dining room and lounge. Everything is smart, bright, minimal, new. They have matching slippers, and arthouse movie posters on the wall, and lo-fi dance music playing from hidden speakers. The windows are blushed with steam from the pans on the stove – a meal on hiatus, prepared but uneaten. His girlfriend cradles a glass of wine on the sofa, her legs tucked underneath her. Something smells of garlic and rosemary. If I wasn't dressed in green, I might be here for dinner. Instead of an oxygen bag and defib, I should be carrying flowers and a bottle of red.

Come and have a seat. Would you like something to drink?

No, thanks.

Some water? A cup of tea?

That's very kind. Why don't you tell me what's wrong?

Normally I'd get some monitoring on – blood pressure, oxygen levels, maybe an ECG – but in Andrew's case I'm confident it can wait a minute or two. He's not sweaty, not pale, not short of breath. There's no distress, discomfort, unease.

I only called for some advice.

999?

He shakes his head.

I never wanted an ambulance. No offence. I looked online, and it said to call 111.

Fine.

So I've got this pain in my shoulder.

He points to his left shoulder.

I've had it a couple of days. The thing is, I think I'm allergic to ibuprofen. I've taken paracetamol. I just wanted to know what else I could take. Like, could I get some codeine or something?

Right.

But I never even got to that bit. They kept asking if the pain went to my chest. If I was feeling sick. How was my breathing? Was I dizzy? They told me to take some aspirin. 'For my shoulder?' I said. 'For the pain in your chest.' 'I don't have any pain in my chest.' That's when they told me you were on the way. I said, 'I really don't think I need an ambulance.'

But here I am.

Here you are.

★

Don't you get sick of all the drunks? Don't the time-wasters drive you mad? Doesn't it get you down when people call you for a nosebleed or a stubbed toe?

These are the slogans. I've heard them many times. It's an inescapable fact: I spend a lot of time with patients who are not very ill.

I could fill this book with the ridiculous calls I've been sent to. Any of my colleagues could. But I suspect it would fast become the dullest book in the world. There might be an initial thrill of exasperation to hear that people call 999 because their thermometer batteries have run out, or they want the housing office to find them new accommodation, or they're worried that their blood pressure is normal today and it's usually high, or because they're in the hospital car park and can't find their way to A&E. But that thrill would last all of half a page before the law of diminishing returns kicked in and a sinking feeling grabbed hold.

It's easy to get frustrated with the abuse of emergency services when that abuse is inflicted from outside. But what about the misuse that comes from within? What if it's intrinsic to the way the system operates?

Andrew's case is a prime example, and far from an isolated one. He doesn't believe he needs an emergency response and hasn't asked for one; he's astonished and embarrassed to have a paramedic in his flat. What's more, he's specifically attempted to use a pathway designed to ease the strain on 999.

The opposite has occurred. What's the result of this and all those similar cases? It's that, as a paramedic, I have a new function: the correction, case-by-case, of repetitive over-caution.

Sometimes I'll go a whole shift without seeing a transporting crew, because no one I encounter needs an ambulance.

Why is this a problem? First, because it's at the root of the ambulance service's struggles with capacity. And second, because somewhere one of the other calls will be for a really sick patient, someone whose life is at risk. And they're still waiting for a response.

Andrew's twenty-eight. He's a young professional without a local GP: he's been too busy to transfer, plus he never gets ill – until now. He describes the pain, locates it, explains what makes it worse. I hook him up to the equipment, check him over. The apparatus breaks the feeling I've just popped round to hang out.

When did it start?

I went climbing Friday. I stretched for a hold and felt a little twinge. When I woke up on Saturday there was a shooting pain across the front of the muscle, here.

Is it worse when you use your arm?

Like a little shock. Just certain movements. To be honest, it feels like I've trapped a nerve or strained the muscle or something. I told them on the phone. But I'm not sure they were following me.

Andrew has an exemplary blood pressure. He takes about eight breaths a minute. His heart rate's 46 – in a good way. The ECG's faultless.

You do a lot of sport?

A bit.

His girlfriend laughs:

You're lucky he's even here!

185

She counts on her fingers: football, climbing, swimming, running. And gym.

You know you've got a slow heart rate?

What is it at the moment?

Forty-six.

That's fast for him.

They've checked it out. It's never been a problem.

The fact is, Andrew's one of the healthiest people I've ever met.

There's an elephant in the back of the ambulance, and it's squeezing the air out of the tyres. Services can tinker at the edges, pushing crews to see more patients, encouraging alternative care pathways, but the biggest challenge of ambulance work remains the persistent dispatch on a massive scale to non-emergency calls. This is the daily reality on the frontline.

Crews get sent to five types of calls:

- *critically ill patients*
- *non-emergency patients who need to go to hospital by ambulance*
- *patients who need an ambulance but not hospital*
- *patients who need to go to hospital, but not by ambulance*
- *patients who do not need either.*

The problem is that the first three categories require an ambulance, but the fourth and especially fifth categories make up the majority of ambulance callouts.

The key question is: why do so many non-emergencies

resemble true emergencies at the telephone stage? It's a complicated issue.

Most emergency calls are made in a state of panic, by people without medical knowledge. They often involve communication barriers and time constraints, and leave little room for in-depth investigation. Plus, there's the central characteristic of the interaction: the call-taker can't see the patient. (This may change in the future.) In short, a wealth of factors that make history-taking in this context challenging.

Yet I would argue that none of these challenges is insurmountable. The creation of sophisticated, nuanced algorithms is perhaps the great endeavour of the IT age.

For example, tonight's call-taker believed Andrew had chest pain – so Andrew received a rapid response and was told to take aspirin, in case he was having a heart attack. Something Andrew said clearly triggered that pathway in the triage system.

Yet to me, the on-scene clinician, there's no suggestion of a heart attack – or even chest pain. One way of eliminating this mismatch would be to audit the two interactions together, to see where and how the initial misunderstanding (or correct diagnosis) occurred, and to find ways it could be avoided (or included) in future. The elimination of all confusion may be impossible, but surely refinements could be made?

I'd say I'm more than 99.9 per cent confident that Andrew is going to be okay. I've taken a full history and assessed everything I can assess. I've excluded all the risk factors I can exclude. But there's always that tiny chance.

If I leave a thousand Andrews at home, with instructions to persist with painkillers and see their GP, eventually one of those Andrews might suffer a catastrophic event. And when he does, I will have been the last healthcare professional to see him. I can't predict the future, but it's not impossible that on that one in a thousand occasion, a certain weariness might have led to a pertinent red flag being missed or undocumented.

The dilemma should arise purely from concern about patient care, but inevitably it's also about organisational accountability, and sometimes individual blame. The obvious solution is to refer everyone onwards, which is a popular tactic in healthcare, but this will result in an extra thousand Andrews – not to mention all the Barrys, Clives, Dereks, Eds and Franks – crowding the waiting areas at A&E. Such a blanket approach is the reason I'm spending my shifts filtering jobs like this in the first place.

There's wisdom in caution, of course, especially when lives might be at stake. But that fear of missing something – of being blamed, of being sued, of being responsible for something terrible – is a double-edged sword. If someone is under-triaged, given the wrong advice or discharged before something goes drastically wrong, the pathway of responsibility – the *cost*, in its multitude of meanings – is easy to trace. But what's harder to trace – yet perhaps far more *costly* in different ways – is the impact on other ill patients, perhaps correctly triaged, of being neglected while responders are redirected to patients whose non-emergency symptoms have, by a linguistic trick or crude assumption, nudged them into a higher-category response.

*

Andrew and his girlfriend are keen to get on with their dinner. They stop short of offering me some, but they'd love to make me a coffee.

No, you're all right, thanks. You go ahead and eat. I'll just go out to my car and write the paperwork.

You can do it here if you want?

So I sit at the table, ticking all the boxes, documenting my diligence, while they eat their aromatic but slightly parched chicken and sip their wine. They ask me some of the standard questions – about stabbings, time-wasters, driving on blue lights – and apologise again for dragging me out. It's really very pleasant.

When I go green back in my car, I'm sent to Mavis, who's been waiting on the floor for three hours with a fractured wrist – because she's a lower priority than a twenty-eight-year-old who pulled a muscle on the climbing wall and wants to know what painkillers to take.

XVIII

The patient is Schrödinger's cat. He's a creature trapped in a box, behind the shroud, out of contact, status unknown. A man in the twilight zone between death and life, where both outcomes are still up for grabs.

I've just made a cup of tea when he drops into my life without warning. Not even finished squeezing the bag when the radio vibrates on my hip.

The job comes down bit by bit. First: a category and a number, the highest level of call, dispatched off the first two questions. It means the caller says the patient's not breathing or breathing noisily. It could be an arrest – or it could be someone who's asleep.

I get to my car as the address completes: the local supermarket. I start the engine – but what to do with the cup of tea? I ditch most of it on the forecourt but keep a few consolation sips in case I'm cancelled. I push en route. Blue lights on. Quick blast of the sirens to make a hole in the traffic. Away I go.

More details land on the screen: thirty-five-year-old male,

reported unconscious, breathing unknown. Typically ambiguous. Apparently collapsed in a toilet cubicle. The caller can't get to him or get a response. Perhaps the patient's had a faint or a fit; perhaps something worse. Perhaps he's just having a few moments' private reflection with his elbows on his knees. I'm not going to know until I get there, so when I pull up across the pavement, I take in everything I can carry: oxygen bag, defibrillator, paramedic bag. It's a long way back to the car.

I weave past waddling shoppers. A washed-out man with a large coat and a Labrador flags me down, phone in hand.

Down here!

He hangs up.

What's happened?

He's not answering. He's in the cubicle.

How long's he been in there?

Ten minutes? Fifteen?

How do you know him?

Well . . .

Is he a friend?

Sort of. Listen, I think he's taken something.

Why do you say that?

It's why he went in.

He holds back the door of the toilets, points at the cubicle –

In there.

– and disappears. I never see him or his dog again.

All is quiet in here. There's a distinct lack of drama. No privacy screens being erected, no store manager keeping customers at bay. An elderly gentleman stands whistling at the urinal; another waits for the wall washer to squirt soap onto his hands. This is not the scene of a critical emergency. Is this a hoax?

The room's three metres square, tiled in beige and lit in yellow and echoing like a cave. It has the customary fragrance of stale urine. The floor looks dry, but that doesn't mean much. There are two urinals, two cubicles, two automatic hand washers and a baby-changing platform. One of the cubicles is closed: I bang on the door.

Hello? Anyone in there?

Do I hear a mumbled reply? No: it's the man at the urinal, groaning in surprise as he turns towards the disturbance. I bang again; no response. I enter the next-door cubicle and stand on the seat to peer over, but then I have second thoughts. What if I crane my head over to see the face of a squatting shopper in the throes of a heroic endeavour? The caller didn't look entirely reliable, and has vanished. Maybe I'm being set up? But I have to investigate. Until that door opens, the cubicle is crammed with all the possible patients, and any and every and no conclusion is still on the cards.

The divider's too close to the ceiling anyway, so I bend down to peer under the door. Is that even worse? The man at the urinal is now openly watching me. I expect to see a pair of shoes and a gather of dropped trousers, but what I actually perceive is a kind of heap – clothing, flesh, material, limbs; it's hard to tell, but it's definitely a human in crisis. Some form of collapse. I'm certain now that I need to get in. I push on the door and bang with purpose –

Hello! Can you hear me? Are you okay in there?

– and then examine the lock. It has a sliding mechanism and shouldn't be hard to force. The hinge opens outwards. I pull out my tough-cut shears, slide them between the door and the cubicle wall, and try to push back the lock. The scissors slide off the smooth metal and make no headway. I try again, but time after time they get no purchase.

Then, out of nowhere, someone from the supermarket café scurries in, slides a butter knife into the lock, releases it in one smooth motion, then pulls it away and scurries back out. Like the caller, he's done his bit and is gone: it's as if he was never there.

The cubicle door swings open. There's the tiny spark of tension. My eyes take in the scene. A tremor of acceleration hits my body: a rapid appraisal and the concurrent formation of a response.

There's a patient who needs help. Big. Heavy. Maybe fifty, maybe thirty. Not sat on the toilet: floored on his knees and bent double between the bowl and the cubicle door. Like a sack, dropped from a height. Bowing down in an unplanned gesture of prostration. I can't see his face, because it's folded forward and sunk into the bulk of his belly.

He's pale. Blue. Grey. Motionless. And not breathing.

There's a small glass bottle or pipe on the floor, some small packets, a syringe. A deduction flashes into my mind: he's taken an overdose of something and collapsed forward, like a punctured inflatable, burying his face in his body mass, suffocating himself in his own flesh.

I shake the patient's shoulder violently and feel for a pulse, but it's no more than a gesture. What I need to do is put him on his back. I grab the thick, floppy wrists, one in each hand, lean back and heave with all my might. His body capsizes forward and slides towards me like butchered meat, and as I drag him from the cubicle I flip him awkwardly at the shoulders and land him supine, slipping a boot under his head to stop it cracking against the tiled floor. Each part of his body slumps outwards to find its lowest point, until he's flat on his back in the middle of the toilet floor.

I pull up the T-shirt, take the pads from the defib, slap them on his chest and turn on the machine. While I watch for the rhythm, I connect a bag-valve mask to the oxygen. The rhythm comes up on the screen: it's slow; it has the shape of a heartbeat but it's too weak to generate a pulse.

I kneel over the patient's head, lace my fingers together, and place my hands, palms down, in the centre of his chest. I lock my elbows, straighten my back, and begin pushing down rhythmically, almost as hard as I can, pushing-and-releasing, pushing-and-releasing, one, two, three, four, five, six, seven, eight, all the way to thirty.

I lift my hands away, take the head, tilt it to lift the nose and chin. I hold the chin with my left hand and grab the bag-valve mask with my right, place the mask over the mouth and nose, and grip it with my thumb and forefinger, pulling the chin up and against the plastic to form a seal, then squeeze twice. The patient's chest lifts, expands, falls, lifts, expands, falls. It's the work of a couple of seconds. I push the priority button on my radio and return my hands to the patient's chest. Again the lock of the elbows, again the brutal downward compressions, again I count to thirty.

My radio buzzes and I update Control: cardiac arrest. The truck's a few minutes away, and they'll send another car. The police are en route too. I squeeze two more breaths, and glance up to see a security guard putting his head in through the toilet door.

Hey! Buddy!

Boss?

Can you give me a hand?

I put my hands back on the chest, push again.

Okay.

Kneel down here for me, next to the patient. We need to work his heart. See how I'm pushing on his chest? I want you to do exactly what I'm doing.

The security guard kneels down between the patient and the cubicle.

Put your hands here. Push down as hard as you can. Just like I'm doing. You push thirty times, same speed as this, then you stop and I put in some air. Okay?

The security guard nods. He places his hands on the patient's chest. He stares at the patient's lifeless face. He only came in to see what all the fuss was about.

I ventilate the patient then tell the security guard to start pushing. I count him through –

One, two, three, four, five –

While he's delivering compressions, I slide a small airway stabiliser into the mouth, to hold the tongue away from the throat.

– Twenty-eight, twenty-nine, thirty. Okay, just stop for a second.

I squeeze in two more breaths.

Okay, and start pushing again. You're doing really well. Just keep doing what you're doing.

The security guard looks shell-shocked, but he's following the instructions, and his compressions are keeping the patient's hopes alive.

The terms *heart attack* and *cardiac arrest* are often conflated. I doubt this patient's had a heart attack, which is death of heart muscle caused by a blockage of the coronary arteries, but he has suffered a cardiac arrest: an absence of circulation to vital organs and specifically the brain, through cessation or critical decline of the heart's pumping action – in practical terms, the lack of a pulse in his neck.

I think the cause here is more likely a breathing failure. Either the drugs have messed with the wiring of his respiratory mechanisms, or they've made him collapse and fatally block his own airway. But the real question is how far down the terminal burrow he's travelled. How long ago did he stop breathing? How much damage has been done? With the right treatment, can he be pulled back out? Or has he gone beyond the point of no return?

By opening the cubicle door, I've answered part of Schrödinger's riddle. But the crucial issue – the patient's survival – is still out for tender. In this sense, the patient's still hidden, still locked away; he's still, potentially, both dead and alive. The real mystery is not what's already happened out of sight, inside the locked cubicle – it's what's still happening right now, out of sight, inside the cells and organs of the patient's body. It's in that hidden realm that I'm attempting to intervene in the name of survival, of preservation, of life.

The police arrive and take over compressions; the security guard disappears like the others, never to be seen again. When the crew turns up there are enough hands to escalate the treatment. We check what we can to rule out other causes, but we treat for an overdose and a shortage of oxygen. I insert a blunt blade into the patient's mouth and lift the tissue of the throat to inspect the airway for foreign bodies, vomit, secretions, anything to inhibit respiration, then insert a rubberised airway device to improve ventilation. One of the crew drills a needle into the patient's shin and administers adrenaline, fluids and naloxone to reverse the effects of what we presume are opiate drugs. Compressions continue throughout.

The reaction to the drugs is almost instant: within two minutes, the patient has a pulse. We stop compressions and mark the time: the magic moment, a return of spontaneous circulation. We've encountered a patient without a pulse, and now he's got one. But it's only part of the story; not by a long way does it mean he's fixed.

We stabilise, check everything, give more naloxone, tidy the scene. Moving the patient is difficult in the confined space, even with multiple helpers. We load him onto the trolley but his arms flop insolently down to the sides; we secure them to the trolley handles to stop them bouncing about. Under the gaze of a small crowd of shoppers, still ventilating with the bag, still monitoring, still ensuring there's a pulse, we wheel him slowly out to the ambulance, ready to transfer to A&E.

As we load the patient on board, his fate hangs in the balance. He's maintaining his circulation, and has responded quickly to treatment, but this is no doubt mainly due to the adrenaline, which can give a positive initial reaction belied by more negative long-term outcomes. We can't yet see the effects of his period of radio silence.

Then, just as we're about to leave, the patient's shoulders lift, his belly sucks in, his chest expands: he's taken a breath on his own. As we stitch our way through the rush-hour traffic, more breaths follow, and I find myself willing him to survive. Of course I do. He's a young man with years left in the world, not a chronically ill patient who's come to the natural end. There are times in this job when, for all its sadness, death feels somehow appropriate because a life has run its course. But there are plenty of others when it's an offence to be battled with, an error that demands opposition.

In polite society, we tend to keep death off to one side. We know it's there, forever looming, but we don't want to give it too much attention in case it gets any ideas. But there are some weeks here when death seems to be everywhere you look.

Initially, you want everyone to survive. This is human nature – and a matter of pride. You think, if you just do your job right, you can amend all those aberrations and keep all those tragedies at bay. Pretty quickly you learn this is not the case: the majority of people who go into cardiac arrest will not make it. It's a brutal truth that takes a hammer to your enthusiasm and puts you firmly in your place, and there's a harsh reality to face: it's not you or what you do; it's just the way it goes. The key is to accept it and persist in doing your best none the less. Death becomes the norm, survival the exception; so you perform your duties and leave the rest to the mystery in Schrödinger's box.

I've never really mastered this skill of accepting the inevitable without a pang of borrowed grief. I can see its benefits; there's a need for vocational detachment, and the less you invest, the fewer catastrophes you take home with a lingering sense of defeat. But I'm not convinced the alternative isn't worse: calm acquiescence to a bleak reality, a psychological surrender that smooths out the peaks and troughs that remind us why we're here. Even now, I'm not sure this voluntary numbness is something I'm ready to accept.

By the time we reach hospital, the patient is breathing for himself – deep animal gasps – and we hand over someone who's technically alive. We've pulled him out of the grave, for now at least. There are grounds for tentative optimism, but it's unclear how long his body went without oxygen – and how much damage this has done.

The target is what's called *survival to discharge* – a patient who walks out of hospital at the end of the process, however long that takes. I hope that will be this patient's future – but I have my doubts. It's a mystery that will only be solved with time – another of Schrödinger's boxes with multiple realities inside.

XIX

How are we doing today, Frank?

I'll tell you upstairs.

Frank spins on his heel, leaves me in the doorway and starts tramping up towards his room.

Why don't you tell me down here?

They're listening, aren't they?

Who?

As if to answer, the manager appears in the doorway:

Oh God, he hasn't called you again, has he?

Don't listen to him! Don't listen to him! He's evil!

I'm here to see Frank, but some information from the manager would help:

Has he already called an ambulance today?

Yesterday. And two the day before. I'm really sorry. Frank, you're supposed to check with us before calling.

Frank stops halfway up the stairs.

Are you coming to check me over or what?

Of course. I'll follow you up.

When I get upstairs Frank is pacing his room, sliding the

200

back of his phone off, on, off, on, off, on. Each time he gets to the window, he flips the blinds open, looks out at the street, left, right, then flips them closed again. More pacing. More sliding the back off the phone and on again. Then the blinds – open, closed. Then more pacing.

So what's wrong, Frank?

Where's the ambulance?

Tell me what's going on and we'll see if we need one.

They're supposed to send an ambulance.

You know how it works, Frank. You need to tell me what's happened.

Huh!

Shoulders hunched, Frank walks back over to the window and looks out.

It should be here by now. I said I had chest pains.

Do you have chest pains?

Maybe.

Frank, listen. They're only going to send an ambulance if we need one.

You mean if you tell them to.

Exactly.

So tell them. I need to go to hospital.

Okay. But why?

I'm entitled to an ambulance. If I call up and say I need an ambulance I'm entitled to get one!

I'm afraid you're stuck with me for now. Let's try and work out what's going on and what we're going to do about it.

You're just standing there chatting! You're not doing your job properly. You're supposed to do stuff. Yeah? Check me. You're

201

supposed to take me to hospital! Right? I don't want to talk about what's going on, I want to go to hospital.

Come and sit down and I'll check you. But, Frank. What do you want them to do for you at hospital? What are we going to say is the problem?

I can't stay here. I don't like the people.

The staff?

And the residents. All of them. They don't like me. They're making me angry. They're stressing me out.

You're feeling upset?

Frank jumps up, opens the fridge door, takes out a bottle of fizzy drink, and takes a great long gulp. He walks back to the window, opens the blind and belches matter-of-factly as he looks left and right.

Frank, do you have anything wrong physically?

I told you!

Do you feel unwell? Do you have any pain?

Frank slumps extravagantly down in the armchair. He takes a deep, theatrical breath. He stares at his phone, then dials a number.

Who are you calling, Frank?

Frank's fingers drum on the arm of the chair.

Frank?

I'm calling an ambulance! Right? I need an ambulance!

I'm already here, Frank.

You're not an ambulance. You're no use to me.

Someone has answered.

Yeah. Hello? Yeah. Right. I need an ambulance. Right?

His foot starts tapping impatiently on the floor. He gives the address.

I've got chest pains. Yeah, pains in my chest, yeah? What?

Frank listens, frowning.

No, he's here . . . No, he came in a car . . . I mean – No . . . He's in front of me . . . What?

Frank holds out the phone.

They want to speak to you.

I take the phone from Frank, identify myself, explain that yes, I'm here, with Frank, and I'm still assessing him, and no, we don't need an ambulance just yet. I thank the call-taker and hang up, hold the phone out to Frank. He snatches the phone without looking.

Right, Frank. Tell me about this chest pain.

Everyone knows Frank. Most people have been to him many times. Those that haven't are familiar with him by reputation instead. Among local crews, like so many of his equivalents all over the country, he sits somewhere between a blot on the occupational landscape and a badge of honour:

Went to Frank three times last week.

We got him two jobs in a row. Left him at home. Drove round the corner and came up green, and we got sent straight back.

Did you take him in?

He's only going to keep calling back, isn't he?

Short, thick-set and bearded, his physique is at odds with the hunched, adolescent way he carries it around. He has the restless impatience of a man conspired against by the world. Beneath the layers of frustration, Frank's recurring complaint is invariably that someone has not done what he wants them to.

He usually calls with chest pains, knowing this is something that can't be ignored, but so far no one's found anything wrong with his heart or his lungs. Not for want of trying: he's one of those patients who might still have the ECG stickers on from a previous encounter, or the cotton wool taped to the crook of his arm where they've just done his bloods. He's younger than me, and physically healthy, and if the NHS still exists in anything like its current form, it's entirely possible that Frank will still be calling multiple ambulances each day in forty years' time.

He's maddening but not malicious. Manipulative but not menacing. Like a dog who never bites but keeps peeing on the carpet, just when you're about to go out, and in full view, as if to send you a message: *I am your responsibility. You cannot ignore me. Don't leave me here alone.* Wilful and unapologetic, but also needy and compulsive. His needs are real, but misdirected.

I spend a lot of my time dealing with people like Frank – more than I ever imagined when I started out. It's the hidden grind of a job where we almost never say no. Perhaps I was naïve not to see this part of the routine coming, but I never imagined a single patient could take up so much of my life – I think I've seen more of Frank this week than I have my own kids. It's perhaps no surprise that nights like this are liable to throw up those age-old questions, which I get asked from time to time: *Am I glad I changed careers? Is this what I expected?*

Would I ever go back? And the less traditional: *What on earth was I thinking, giving up a nice comfy job in an office – to do this?*

At times like this, I consider the crushing effect on any kind of social life of shift work, where evenings rarely exist in any meaningful sense. But then I balance this against the very practical ways it can help with childcare. There's the cherished opportunity of days off when others are at work – of doing the school run or being the only viewer in the cinema's morning showing, or supermarket shopping with the weekday mafia of the retireds. But there's also the encroaching facsimile of a family dynamic where, in effect, two single parents share a dwelling, a bed and kids – but not always a life.

When I'm at work, I might appreciate the freedom to be out and about, and even drive on the wrong side of the road from time to time – but contrast that privilege with the fact I've got up at four-thirty in the morning to be there and will spend most of my day trying to work out where I'm going to go for my next wee.

Of course, these are the standard appraisals of any occupation, the kinds of thing anyone could supply themselves. However, I suspect that when my friends ask me if I'm glad I made the switch, they're after a bit more nuance in terms of emotional and psychological fulfilment; I suspect what they really want to know is: do I now feel more satisfied, more complete than I did before?

The simple answer, as I'm sure it would be for almost anyone, is that it depends when you ask. When I've just arrived at the cath-lab with a patient who's had a cardiac arrest in the workplace but is now alive and breathing and about to have their heart fixed, then I'd have to say that I feel pretty pleased to be here. You'd be hard pressed to improve on this moment for pure job satisfaction. On the other side of the coin, when it's seven o'clock on a Sunday morning and I'm cycling home in the wind and rain after a thirteen-hour shift spent dealing with the aggressive, the argumentative, the inebriated and the worried well, and all I can think about is my friends who made very different life choices and aren't even awake yet in their cosy beds, then I have been known to rehearse the last of those enquiries – *just what was I thinking?* – on silent repetition in my brain.

You gotta move me.

   What do you mean?

   This place. Yeah? You gotta move me out.

   Move where?

   Back to the old place.

   Why's that, Frank?

   They're not looking after me.

   Who?

   The staff. The staff here!

   Looking after you how?

   They're stressing me out. They're not cooking my meals.

   Are they supposed to cook your meals?

   And they're always asleep, right?

   They're not asleep now. I just saw them downstairs.

   You're not here for them!

   I know.

Why do you always take their side?

No one's taking sides, Frank. When are they asleep?

In the night.

Right.

When I get stressed.

Frank, this is supported living. They're not supposed to cook your meals.

You're not listening to me, yeah? I want to go back to the old place.

Was it better there?

Yeah. They looked after me better.

So why did you move?

They chucked me out.

Why did they do that?

I was abusive to the staff.

Okay.

He just comes out with this. Doesn't try to sugar the pill.

So . . . Were you violent?

He shakes his head.

I swore at them and shouted. Yeah? And broke some things.

Last time I came to Frank, I arranged a cab to take him to A&E. It was night-time and winter and patients were waiting hours for crews to turn up. Frank was anxious and upset and wanted to see a doctor. He took the taxi to the hospital, then walked home and called 999 again. He told the next paramedic he had to go in by ambulance.

I don't feel safe in a cab.

Why's that?

What if something happens on the way?

What d'you think's going to happen?

Anything could happen! I don't feel safe!

Most people would spin these stories to win over the listener. But not Frank. Frank's candour is revealing. It seems that shame is not a problem for Frank. So it's also not a constraint on his behaviour. He displays no embarrassment while revealing that he was abusive to the people who look after him, just as he shows no embarrassment about walking home from the hospital to call another ambulance to take him straight back. These are not things that need to be defended or explained. They're more like supporting evidence in his ongoing plea.

Why were you abusive, Frank?

They weren't doing their job. It was making me angry.

Isn't that the same problem as here?

No! It was better there. My room was next to the office. I could call them.

In the night? When you were stressed?

Here they don't care. They don't do anything! I could be dying, they don't care.

Do you call them a lot?

Only when I need them.

But the office is downstairs?

You just saw them, didn't you? You just spoke to them downstairs! When I go to hospital, I'm going to tell them. They've gotta move me back to the old place.

You know they're not going to do that, don't you, Frank?

Well somewhere new then.

Frank. That's not what A&E is for. They can't help with that.

What are you going to do then?

Me?

Yeah. You. What are you going to do? I've got chest pains.

I've checked you over, Frank. There's nothing abnormal.

My chest is tight. Really tight, yeah? I feel like, if you don't call me an ambulance, something really bad might happen.

Like what?

I don't know. Something bad.

Why don't we have a chat with the manager?

Chat, chat, chat! That's all you people ever do!

I know. It's tiresome, isn't it? I'm sorry, Frank. Who are you calling now?

Frank has his phone out again.

Hello, Marvin? Hello? Oh. Where's Marvin? Right, who's that then? Yeah? I need to be moved out. Tonight. You've gotta move me back to the old place. I'm not spending another night here. I need to be moved now. I've got the paramedics here. I'm not well. I'm getting chest pains. I'm getting worked up, yeah? I feel like something bad's gonna happen. Someone needs to sort this out.

The conversation with Marvin's substitute – a social worker, it seems – travels the same roads we've already been down: the well-worn highways of Frank's grievances, the roundabouts of alternative solutions he won't consider, the blind cul-de-sacs of his determination, and finally the emergency stops when he doesn't get the answer he wants and bails out of the conversation, putting the phone down or storming off, like a stuntman diving out of a moving vehicle. This time it's the social worker, but it could easily be his cousin, his dad, his GP, his support worker. He's in search of an ally, someone to validate him, but tonight no one's playing ball.

Frank is surrounded by people attempting to help him cope with the challenges of his life – yet nothing anyone does is enough. Most of his interactions, in fact, are with people who have some degree of responsibility for him. In one sense, he's immensely fortunate that this network exists. But it's also possible to see the crippling effects of institutionalisation. He's become almost entirely dependent on other people, and his own responsibilities have almost disappeared. The fact he rarely has to create anything, nurture anything, contribute anything, earn anything, means he has no investment in the basic give-and-take of human contact. He's like a child who doesn't have to grow up, and he doesn't know any different.

It's this mismatch that I find so gruelling. Give me a cardiac arrest any day of the week, because those metaphorical cul-de-sacs and roundabouts are starting to feel incredibly real. It's like the fatigue at the end of a really long journey – except that on this excursion, when you pull over and turn off the ignition, you find you're back where you started. I want to engage with Frank more productively, to have some kind of impact, but it doesn't seem to work this way: all expressions of concern are simple fuel to the flames. You can't take him to task for anything, because he doesn't show any ambition for change.

I'm starting to worry about my supply of patience. Could it be in terminal decline? These encounters are supposed to be water off a duck's back. Plenty of my colleagues have made their peace with this part of the job, and speak with affection about the frequent callers – even if they know, deep down, that these jobs are a long way from our intended purpose. I can see how that makes for an easy life; I'm just not sure I can keep going round and round that circuit.

I think of the times when I've spent hours coaxing and helping a difficult patient, the mental energy I've expended, and how drained I feel at the end. I think about the following day, when I've switched roles and put on my domestic hat, and then discovered a complete lack of patience when my kids have told me I've bought the wrong bread, and they no longer eat cheese, and today they're going to go to school in bare feet or not at all. I think about how I've thrown a little tantrum of my own, and feel ashamed at the disparity between its source and its target. Do I really have no patience left for the people whose welfare is more than just a professional concern? Heaven forbid that something real might happen in my own life and that tantrum might be directed at a patient one day. Then where would I be? I wonder if these are the simple fluctuations of a so-called caring vocation – or is this a more permanent, debilitating character shift? And, if so, is it a sacrifice I'm willing to make?

If this were a novel, there'd be some kind of resolution. A moment of insight for both Frank and me. Not a transformation, but a lesson, a change, a hope.

Life, however, can be relentless. We both stick to our guns, until Frank bails out.

Forget it. Forget the whole thing. I'm going out.

Okay, Frank. If that's what you want.

I'll see you again.

I'm sure you will.

XX

Aside from major road crashes, the ambulance calls that pro-
voke the most curiosity, reverence and unease in the general
public are stabbings and shootings. It's easy to see why.
They're the calls where paramedics get to be the version of
themselves they've seen on TV – the version that doesn't
really exist in the day-to-day. They're the calls that colleagues
will ask about tomorrow, the calls that might appear on the
news.

Violent assaults fulfil the classic requirements of fascination
and dread. Anxiety about their prevalence in contemporary
society, about the senselessness of young deaths, about their
possible links to gangs, drugs, organised crime, deprivation
and inequality, and of course about the possibility of someone
we know getting caught up in them, only add to the sense of
shock and awe.

Yet, for ambulance crews in certain areas, I have to be
honest: knife and gun incidents can quickly become quite
run-of-the-mill. Initially they feel like a big deal, because
they're outside most people's experience. But before long, a

sense of repetition, dare I say it, of routine begins to take hold. Perhaps this is because the drama and the response are often disproportionate to the severity of the injury: an armada of emergency vehicles flies to the scene to find someone with a cut on their arm. Perhaps it's because, even when the injuries are serious, we rarely give much treatment: oxygen, dressing, IV cannula, rapid transfer to a suitable hospital. It's all over in the blink of an eye.

Stabbings and shootings may carry the trappings of contemporary turmoil: the flutter of the police cordon, the echo of sirens and the glare of blue lights. But they soon become just part of the ebb and flow of the emergency landscape.

The description on the screen is uncharacteristically clear:

UNKNOWN AGE MALE. GUNSHOT WOUND.
NOT BREATHING

It takes me by surprise. I read it twice. There's not much room for doubt.

I'm on an ambulance and we're halfway through the night. We've been pottering about for the first half of the shift, dropping patients to A&E, referring others to their GPs. We haven't broken sweat, and I'd have bet any money that's how the rest of the night would play out. But it just goes to show, when you press that green button, you never know what's coming next.

We're two miles away. It's a local night-spot with a reputation for trouble. A crossroads of cultures and postcodes. We're given an RVP, or rendezvous point, at a safe distance of a few hundred metres. We make our way there and wait with another crew and a car for permission to approach.

This is always a strange hiatus. Something very bad has happened and someone urgently needs our help. We're primed, restless, ready to get involved. But we wait in our vehicles for someone to take us off pause. A breezy pop song plays on the radio. People walk past and give us curious looks. *Why aren't they with a patient? I thought the ambulances were rushed off their feet . . .*

We see flashing blue lights in the distance. A minute later we get the message:

POLICE ON SCENE. PLEASE COME FORWARD

The FRU and the other crew bolt away at speed. My crew-mate and I follow at the rear.

The scene glows with the lights from the nearby takeaways and off-licences. The street's awash with police and bystanders being pushed back as we arrive. This is an unfolding situation. We find the patient up a side street, between the rows of parked cars. A police van has parked across the junction – blocking the road and shedding some light on the gloomy scene.

There's a lot of noise: screaming, crowd control, a relentless banging sound from further up the road. My colleagues kneel around the patient, in the middle of the tarmac, under the flickering blue light. One of the officers pushes on his chest. First-aid kits, medic bags and oxygen bottles are laid out in a crude circle. His clothes are being cut off as we arrive. There's very little blood.

Our colleague on the car has arrived just seconds before us, but has already applied the pads and set up the BVM. The job is 'as given', the patient not breathing.

We've got a PEA rhythm. Workable rhythm but I can't feel a pulse. There's some blood in the mouth. Can someone grab the suction?

Someone passes it across. The officers from the armed response unit tell us what they know:

This is where he dropped.

Maybe two shots, we're not sure yet.

When we got to him, he wasn't breathing.

We put him on his back, opened his airway, started CPR.

One of my colleagues takes over chest compressions. The FRU stays at the head end:

Can someone pass me my airway roll? I'm going to put in an iGel. Can someone get access?

I grab my cannula roll and kneel at the right arm.

Has someone reported to the trauma team?

Doing it now. They're five minutes away.

I wrap a tourniquet around the patient's bicep and there's a prominent vein in the crook of the arm. I select the biggest cannula I've got, thinking he might need some blood when the trauma team arrive – we don't yet know the definitive injuries – then clean the arm and slide the cannula into the vein. I cap it, flush it, tape it down, then run a bag of fluids through a giving set, attach it and open up the catch so the fluids flow. I hold the bag out to one of the officers:

You mind being a drip stand?

He takes the bag. The medic at the head secures the airway

device and listens with a stethoscope: air's going into both lungs. Then it's time to analyse the heart rhythm.

Everyone stop for a second. Quick rhythm check.

We stare at the screen. The banging noise is still going on.

Okay, there's a rhythm on the screen. Can we feel for a pulse?

Three-point pulse check, guys.

Anything?

Nothing carotid. Femoral? Radial?

We're having to shout to be heard.

Nope.

Nope.

Okay. Let's carry on.

Hang on, guys. Just before we start again. Shall we sit him up and check his back?

So we grab an arm, a shoulder, the head, and lift him to a sitting position, and quickly check his back for injuries.

All clear. Nothing there.

Good. Back down again. And let's carry on.

The compressions recommence.

I know nothing about this patient, and I'm happy to keep it that way. I can see that he's young, maybe early twenties, healthy-looking, with a life ahead. I barely look at his face, because that's not going to help. I don't need to know if he has siblings, or children of his own; if he's at college or an aspiring musician; if he's been caught up in a case of mistaken identity, or targeted by association – or if he's well known to the police.

This is the cold trajectory of frontline endurance: keeping

reality at arm's length. No names are needed; no details pertain. Few calls better illustrate the psychological gap between emergency response and 'normal' life than a stabbing or a shooting – and I'm not sure the comparison shows us in a great light. If we were trying to upset ourselves, we'd find specifics to relate to, look for ways to identify, consider the tragedy of it all. Yet the tendency instead is to avert the eyes from the familiar details – to do the opposite of empathise – because when the dramatic signifiers are stripped away, there's still a patient to care for like any other.

Is there something heartless about this reaction? Are we just being pragmatic – or denying ourselves a basic human response? Do we really care so little about the person we're treating? If I was starting to worry about the numbing effects of this job on the mindset of the emergency responder in general, and myself in particular, then this was an obvious place to start – because something was happening that I had never expected. I had been on my voyage of exposure beyond the normal boundaries, been to places and seen things I'd not imagined before. I was more informed now about many of the things that go on in the world, but also somehow less hopeful, perhaps a less positive person. And now I worried I was being reworked – as a callous distortion of my former self, a version who, in spite of my best intentions, was becoming blasé about death.

Suddenly the scene is calm.

Treatment is still going on, but there's a new sense of composure. The incessant banging has stopped, and the sudden silence reminds me how stressful noise can be. This has coincided with the arrival of the trauma team – two jumpsuited doctors, a paramedic and an observer. Their air of experience and authority has brought its own infusing serenity: they take everything in order and without shock or alarm. And then there's the fact that, at the last rhythm check, the patient had a pulse.

This means we've stopped resuscitating and are preparing to move – but it's not the triumphant moment it might be. Things still look very bleak. If the patient's injuries were different, there'd be more we could do. A massive blood loss would require volume replacement and wound repair. A penetrating injury in the chest might demand a needle decompression – a therapeutic puncture wound to release air that's trapped in the pleural space and restricting the inflation of the lungs and the major circulation. In the most serious cases, the trauma doctor might open up the chest and attempt some rapid roadside surgery, in a place that's about as far from an operating theatre as you can get. These are the last-ditch, critical treatments made when death's getting the upper hand and something exceptional needs to be done – but none of them is indicated here: all we can do is stabilise and transport to the trauma centre for further care.

The trauma team intubate the patient and we move him to the ambulance for transportation. The emphasis is on methodical efficiency, not a desperate rush. He still has a pulse, so the resuscitation element has been successful so far, but this hasn't corrected the initial problem, the one that put him into cardiac arrest in the first place, the damage that the bullet has done.

As they close the doors of the ambulance and pull away

on lights, I doubt this patient is going to survive. It's another young life cut short in the gloomy banality of a street attack, not by a biological failure or a freak occurrence, but by the casual choice of another human being. When did ending a life get to be so mundane?

As I write this, knife and gun crime are once again headline news. After a recent spate of fatal stabbings, politicians and law-enforcers have been trading public statements, and various interested parties have passed comment on the complex causes of such crimes, and the thorny questions of what can and should be done.

For the emergency services and the trauma hospitals, these violent assaults are something of a gloomy constant, a normalised outrage that keeps on coming – but with occasional fluctuations and what feels like an inexorable upward trend. Often, we're told, these spikes of activity occur when related incidents or retaliatory attacks follow each other.

Much of this passes by in the background of public awareness, perhaps with minor news reports and localised concern. There's a consensus that, although it's happening on our streets and in our towns and cities, it's mainly restricted to a subculture of gangs and drugs and even shady rites of passage. I've sometimes been to a serious assault of an evening and expected to see a news report the following day, only to find it hasn't warranted a passing mention, and wondered why it didn't qualify. Yet from time to time, a kind of tipping point of indignation is reached, as one crisis overlaps with another and the weight of repetition seems to demand a response.

Media coverage and wider disquiet are obviously stirred by the increasing frequency and fatality of attacks. But it's not just about numbers: I also sense that the levels of exposure and concern relate to the types of attacks and the victims who are targeted – and what this says about how close the problem has come to what we might call the mainstream. Incidents that bear the signs of gang skirmishes or ongoing rivalries may be cause for worry, but they don't appear to generate the shock of an attack that intrudes on a more traditional and widespread public experience. In other words, we seem to concern ourselves more about some victims than others.

There's something disturbing about this tendency, because it implies a kind of victim hierarchy. Yet we can probably recognise it as a fairly standard human response. Whether we attribute it to prejudice, shared experience, some kind of media bias, or the out-workings of our own unspoken assumptions, what lies at the root of this phenomenon is surely simple self-preservation. We are determining whether these incidents are something we need to worry about as interested but distant observers – or as people who might one day be subject to their effects. Bad news gets worse, the closer it comes to home.

The paradox here is that we feel reassured when there's a link to illegality, because that connection provides an explanation and takes the danger that little bit further away from our front doors. We can tell ourselves we're safe, because we're not involved in the world these incidents occur in, and don't intend to be if we can possibly help it.

In many ways, this is the same process that emergency responders go through. Faced with the consequences of casual slaughter and routine violence, the easy way to deal with all that bloodshed is to put it in a box with a simple, unambiguous label. So much of this stuff is just too close for comfort: it's happening on the streets where we live or work, or where our kids catch the bus to school or our parents walk to the pharmacy or the corner shop. We need an explanation to cling onto, or we'd never leave the house.

So if we hear informally that an attack looks gang-related, or that the victim is well known locally for all the wrong reasons, then we grab hold of that information with both hands. It makes us feel a bit safer and allows us to carry on.

Of course, in the long run, you have to wonder at the effects of this wilful detachment. You have to wonder if it's good for our perception of the world, our engagement with our fellow humans, our sense of wrong and right, and, ultimately, our own mental health.

XXI

There's something in the act of calling an ambulance that seems to release the inner puppy in a large portion of the British public. It's in equal parts entertaining, maddening and strangely reassuring. High on the thrill of participation in an emergency scenario, apparently rational individuals are liable to begin bouncing about excitedly, yapping their helpful suggestions and describing their own involvement in great detail, as if they're expecting to have their tummies rubbed or receive a marrow-based treat.

When I'm called to an unconscious female in the early afternoon, I'm in little danger of missing the location, because she's collapsed outside a busy local railway station. Nevertheless, as I round the bend on the approach, I'm greeted with the sight of a grown woman, leaping about in the bus lane of a busy road and describing enormous circles with both arms. Even when it's clear I've seen her, the pantomime shows no sign of relenting; rather, as if she's on the runway at Heathrow, she employs an exaggerated bilateral chopping motion with her hands to tell me where to park.

Admittedly, there are times when I'd be grateful to have the way clearly shown. Finding unmarked flats in high-density developments at three in the morning is one of the trials of working alone on the car. But when someone gets so caught up in their good Samaritan role that they begin hopping like Tigger in the stream of rush-hour traffic, it suggests there's going to be more to deal with than just a patient. It feels like that moment when your mum waves across the busy school playground, calling your name ever louder and more piercingly when you don't respond. And, in just the rebellious fashion any self-respecting youngster would adopt in that situation, I have to admit that I now follow standard practice, if not official policy, by driving past the woman trying so ardently to flag me down and pulling up ten yards further down the road.

Before I've turned off the engine, she's alongside the car and has opened the driver's door.

Didn't you see me? I was waving.

Oh, yes. Thank you. I wanted to leave some space for the ambulance.

Aren't you the ambulance?

The big ambulance.

Oh. I see. Well. She's over here. She seems to be breathing, but she won't wake up.

Okay, just let me get my things.

I go to the boot.

Wow! You have so much to carry. It's like a mobile hospital, isn't it? Can I help with something?

Thank you.

223

I hand her the lightest of three bags, and she scurries off towards the patient, while I follow behind with more measured strides. Ambulance crews work tirelessly at not looking too keen – indeed, for some it's perhaps the aspect of the job at which they most excel – but it's not simply for the sake of appearances that crews so rarely break into a run: staying composed when perhaps a dozen bystanders are yelling excited suggestions is as much a matter of studied demeanour as it is innate sangfroid. As ever with this job, it's a case of playing the part.

The patient is flat on her back on the paved concourse outside the station, guarded by three bystanders and my new assistant. Each of them has the full-bladdered restlessness of people keen to look helpful. Meanwhile, the tide of travellers flows past in both directions, relieved that someone else has broken their schedule to do the right thing.

The first thing I spot is the patient's chest moving up and down. That's good, at least. The second is the two overflowing holdalls beside her, and her thick coat and several layers of clothes, despite it being a warm summer afternoon. I put down my bag and the defib and kneel at her side, feeling for a pulse at her wrist.

Is she okay?

What do you think's wrong?

Did we do the right thing?

What are you doing?

I can't believe people were just walking past!

Is there something we can do?

You are going to help her, aren't you?

She's probably younger than I am, but the ordeals of her life, transcribed on her face like a life-story encrypted in abrasions and wounds, give her the look of someone much older. She is slim to the point of scrawniness and pale, with greasy, thinning hair and gaps in her teeth. Grey smudges can be seen on her neck and jaw, as if she's been dusted for fingerprints, and her left cheekbone bears the yellow after-thought of a black eye. Her hands are grubby, her cracked fingernails encrusted with dirt, her slender forearm decorated with bruises and assorted scars – all clues as to what's occurred today.

Tell us what's going on. Please.

Two of my welcoming committee have seen their chance to leave, but the other pair are too heavily invested to move on just yet. They watch my every move.

I pinch the patient's earlobe, depress her nailbed with my pen, squeeze the flesh above her shoulder, but there's no response. Her breathing is a shuddering afterthought. I can't smell alcohol, can't see any fresh injury.

Aren't you going to do something?

Aren't you going to help her?

I glance up at them.

Sorry?

You don't seem to be doing very much.

Some days this would get my goat. I'd be muttering in my head on the theme of the ill-informed bystanders. Cursing their excitable altruism and its consequent hindrances, all the while smiling thinly and thanking them for their help. No one knocks on the cockpit door and offers to fly the plane just because of a bit of turbulence. But crowd control forms a decent part of ambulance life, and today I'm able to see this maddening enthusiasm for what it is: a group of worried individuals caught up in the drama of the moment, urged on by each other, projecting their concern onto the rather dishevelled responder who's answered their call. I can't say I blame them: I'm a pretty disappointing version of the heroic rescuer they imagined. But all is not lost. I'm about to make their day.

Right, ladies. I'm going to need your help. Is that okay?

They both nod briskly in reply.

Of course, of course.

Just tell us what to do.

It would be easy to bite back, but the better option is to make them feel useful.

Can you help me get her on her side?

Granted a great honour, they kneel tentatively beside the patient, watching what I do to make sure they don't fluff their lines. Between the three of us we roll the patient onto her right side to face me, bending her legs and arms into a stick-man running pose so that she doesn't roll back. Her limbs are floppy, pliable like plasticine.

Can you pull her arm out of the jacket for me? Good. And fold it round behind her and under her head? The jacket, not the arm . . . Perfect.

I push her jaw open and slide a curved airway protector over her tongue, twisting it into place. It sits in the back of the throat, hooking her tongue out of harm's way.

You're stopping her from swallowing her tongue?

Sort of, yes.

226

The fact she tolerates this intrusion, doesn't cough or push it out, means she's out for the count.

Okay. Pass me that bag, please.

I remove a clear mask, connect it to the oxygen, strap it round the patient's head so that it straddles her mouth and nose, then take a second packet, this one a nasal cannula, plug it into the defib, then hook it under her nose and around her ears, a tiny flap of plastic overlapping her lips, to give me a rapid visual measurement of her breathing.

Can you hold up her arm?

I wrap the cuff around and push the BP. I snap the oxygen probe on her finger, check the temperature in her ear and the blood sugar on her finger. I explain what I'm doing as I go along, and find to my surprise that, rather than distracting or delaying me, the verbalisation helps me streamline my actions. Likewise, my helpers seem reassured. No – more than reassured: they look exhilarated.

So what do you think's wrong with her?

Well . . .

I'm reluctant to be specific.

. . . There's a number of possibilities.

We thought it might be a heroin overdose?

Oh . . . Right . . .

Having hedged my bets, I've had my thunder stolen.

It's just – we both watched that Ambulance *programme last week. On TV. Did you see it?*

No . . .

It was very good.

I might have been working . . .

227

You should watch it.

Yes, I probably should.

It was very educational.

Was it?

I'm sure it's on iPlayer.

I take out the drugs pack and break the seal. I fish around for a needle.

Some of the people they had to deal with!

Oh. Wasn't it frustrating?

Completely!

These two are going to be lifelong friends.

Anyway, there was a man on there, a bit like this.

I take a vial from the drugs pack.

And he'd taken an overdose.

Heroin.

It was terrible.

Do you think that's what this is?

My eyes are on the patient.

I'd say there's a good chance.

Really?

Wow . . .

To say they're pleased with this endorsement of their theory would be an understatement. Notwithstanding that there's an unconscious woman between them, they look at each other with open delight. But that's not the end of it. Buoyed by the success of their diagnostic instincts, they now take a leap into the treatment side of the scenario.

So . . .

Yes?

Does that mean you're going to give her the Narcan?

I'm just about to snap the vial. Of, yes, the Narcan.

I beg your pardon?

Are you going to give her the Narcan? Isn't that what it's called? Narcan?

I'm sure that's what they called it on the TV.

It was! They gave him the Narcan and he woke up.

Did they?

They injected it.

Then he woke up and swore at them and walked off.

Are you going to give her the Narcan?

Has it really come to this? I'm used to dealing with windmilling philanthropists on the roadside. I'm accustomed to spontaneous experts at the scene of car accidents. I've learnt to smile patiently when family members criticise my methods. I've even had some practice at explaining that I'm not trying to poison the patient, simply offering them something to help with the pain.

But never before have I been told by a member of the public which drug I should give.

And people say TV's not educational . . .

Once I've administered the injection, I have a quick look for alternative causes – and not only to show there's more to this lark than watching a couple of documentaries and being in the right place at the right time. Any proud tradesperson likes to keep something to themselves, but there may well be something else going on. Yet everything points to the amateurs hitting the jackpot first time: the patient's pupils are tiny, and I find what looks like a small crack pipe in her coat pocket; plus, when I examine her arms with a cannula in mind, it's clear these veins have carried a lot of hypodermic traffic in the past.

The ambulance crew arrives and I run them through what's occurred. We keep the new recruits involved in lifting the patient onto the bed, and it's at this moment that the much-celebrated Narcan (naloxone) suddenly works its magic: the patient coughs out the airway, opens her eyes, looks around wildly and, reaching down to her pocket without missing a beat, grabs a sandwich and begins stuffing it ravenously into her mouth. We try to take it from her, but she is suddenly mighty; she pushes us away and gobbles down more lunch. As we're moving her to the ambulance she gradually slips back into her original torpor, and by the time she's on board she's unresponsive again, but this time with a mouthful of congealed bread.

The medic from the truck uses his forceps to pull several large globules of partially chomped dough out of the patient's mouth, saliva string stretching as he dumps them in the waste. He suctions the attendant spittle and positions the airway to keep it open, while we give a further dose of the as-seen-on-TV Narcan. The crew prepares to transport the patient to A&E.

When I get off the ambulance to let them go, I'm met with two wide-eyed faces outside the back door, eager for an update. If they had tails, they'd surely be wagging. But all they want is to know their sacrifice has been worthwhile.

Thanks for your help, ladies. I couldn't have done it without you.
Perhaps it's a matter of perspective. On the one hand,

they've brought a premature end to the patient's hard-earned escapism and ruined her day: she won't thank them for it. On the other, they've made sure she'll still be here tomorrow – perhaps for someone else to do the same again. Ultimately, they've only done what anyone would want done for them: gone the extra mile for a human being in need. And I can't blame them for that – it's what this job is all about.

XXII

It's the early hours of the morning, and the front door's open. It's unclear if this is in obedience or defiance of a laminated poster inside the entrance:

TO ALL RESIDENTS!!
PLEASE COULD NO ONE **ALWAYS** MAKE
SURE THEY LEAVE MAIN DOOR OPEN.
THANKS!!

There's no one around. I follow the police officers inside. There's blood on the floor, a shiny brown linoleum that's probably designed to hide such spillages, but these drips still have a fresh, glossy sheen. The trail leads up the stairs.

Hello? Hello?

No one responds.

It's a large Edwardian townhouse that's been broken down into one-room flats and crammed with anonymous strangers who only come out when the coast is clear. Every door has a heavy lock and a stack of unclaimed post sits in the hallway; the gloss of the communal woodwork has turned yellow and there's a permanent aroma of cooking oil in the air. Other instructional posters have been taped to the woodchip walls, telling residents not to play aloud music, to make sure they sort their rubbishes properly, and what to do if there's a fire.

We follow the line of drips up the stairs. A smudged brown handprint on the door of Room 4 tells us where we need to go, so the officers knock and try the handle.

The door opens to reveal a home in a box. An electric heater commands the centre of the room, a tiny kitchen unit stands against the far wall, a bedside lamp illuminates the carpet in one corner. On a crumpled mattress on the floor, cross-legged, bald and shirtless, a Buddha on a hunger strike, sits James: a skinny man in his thirties pressing a scrunched-up, bloodied T-shirt against his left forearm. He looks up at us like a boy who's wet his pants in class.

I'm really sorry, fellas.

James lifts the wadded T-shirt to reveal his lacerated arm. He has cut himself about a dozen times with a razor, overlaying a dense network of glossy old scars with a lattice of new wounds. They are raw, angry and encrusted with freshly bobbled clots.

When I ask about the blade he's used, he nods at a wooden chair doubling as a table, where a brand new razor, stained with a narrow triangle of blood, sits on the top of its packaging.

Is this the only one?

He nods.

Do you mind if we check?

233

He stands to let the officers have a good look around, then sits back down.

You did all this yourself, James?

He nods.

Have you cut yourself anywhere else?

He shakes his head.

Have you taken any tablets? Done anything else to hurt yourself?

No.

Okay. How are you feeling, mate?

Pretty stupid.

Can you tell me what happened?

James shrugs.

Same as always. Few drinks. Feeling shit. Can't sleep. Cut my arm. Nothing new.

How much've you had to drink?

Four cans.

Any drugs?

A shake of the head.

I examine the cuts. Most are superficial and have already clotted, but a few of them are deep enough to need closing up. James can see what I'm thinking.

I'm not going to A&E.

Right.

I'm telling you that now.

Let's have a look at these wounds. They might need some proper attention.

I don't want to mess you around, mate. I respect what you do. But I'm not going to go.

★

What's happened to James tonight is neither new nor extraordinary, and he's not interested in pretending otherwise. He doesn't try to transfer the drama, doesn't play games or spin us a yarn. While I clean and dress the wounds, he stares at his shoes and tells us, plainly, how it is.

He suffers with depression and drinks every day, doesn't work or see his family, and has few friends. He's been taken into hospital under section in the past, has a long history of self-harm, and sees a community mental-health nurse every fortnight. These are the simple facts that summarise his life in fifty words: the resumé of a stock character from the neighbourhood where health and social care don't quite overlap. His predicament is not uncommon; it's the kind of story you might hear as background colour on a radio news feature any afternoon of the week.

Of course there's more to it than that. James has some solid, uncomplicated insight into his problems, even if that insight has not released him from its shackles. He talks plainly and without self-pity about the damage his behaviour has done.

Is there someone we can call?

He shakes his head, fiddles with his laces.

Family?

Nope.

Friends?

Nope.

There must be someone, James.

My mum would've been the one.

Shall we give her a call?

He shakes his head.

She wouldn't answer.

She doesn't want to speak to you?

Something like that.

What if we call from a different phone?

She'd know. Even without answering.

When did you last see her?

She's put up with a lot of shit from me. This has been going on a long time.

Let's at least give it a try.

No. She's got her own problems. She doesn't need all this.

He waves his hand at his current situation. He's candid about his drinking – how he feels reliant on it, has given up many times in the past and sometimes wishes he could stop, but other days it's his only friend. Now, in his thirties, he sees this as who he is.

They've put a lot of effort into getting me sober.

Who has?

Everyone. Support workers. Family. You people. The doctors.

Been in the system a while?

Can't say I haven't had a chance.

That doesn't mean you can't have another.

He shakes his head.

There's other people. It's their turn now.

And about A&E he is adamant:

They don't know what to do with people like me.

What do you mean?

They'll put me in a room for six hours. No one will talk to me. Then, when I'm just about to walk out, someone will come in and ask all the questions I've been asked a hundred times before. They call it a place of safety. All they're interested in is making sure I don't kill myself. Something you learn pretty quick about mental health. No one wants anything to do with you.

The sad truth is, he's right. More and more of our calls revolve around mental-health crises. Yet the emergency medical system is set up to manage physical problems, and in my experience the provision for psychiatric patients, especially 'out of hours', lags way behind. There's been much public hand-wringing about provision for mental health recently, along with promises of funding and services. Some things seem to be improving. But anyone encouraged by such reports should try to access help for a patient who's self-harming at midnight: they'll almost always be sent to A&E. And, as James and so many others explain, A&E is the last place that patient wants to be. As a result, mental-health patients, often at their lowest ebb, can feel as if the people treating them would be more comfortable dealing with someone else.

Are such attitudes evident in ambulance crews? I hope not. What I suspect most crews feel about psychiatric calls is something closer to trepidation – about dealing with something that veers outside our scope of expertise – and frustration we can't do more to help.

Mental-health calls often have a twin focus: the immediate physical manifestation – overdose, self-harm, chest pains – and the more profound, psychological issue behind it. Although there's a reservoir of emotional and social complexity beneath the reason for the call, the physical element normally takes priority. Patients who've taken an overdose or self-harmed will need medical treatment and clearance before psychiatric services can begin; mental-health teams will not even see patients under the influence of alcohol or drugs. This inevitably delays, or even prevents, access to the part of the system that's going to be of most benefit.

It may come as no surprise that ambulance crews are more comfortable dealing with the physical emergency than the underlying psychiatric or emotional crisis. People in emergency medicine, both in and out of hospital, are used to fixing things. We identify problems and implement solutions, and temperamentally we're used to seeing results. We like to think of ourselves as interveners, counter-attackers, crisis-resolvers; we pride ourselves on being people of action rather than anguish.

For creatures who like to keep things simple, this means addressing problems with a logical set of priorities. If one treatment doesn't work, we move on to the next. Asthma attack? Nebulise some salbutamol. Not helping? Add atrovent and set off for hospital. Still suffering? Give some hydrocortisone and put on the lights. No improvement? Move on to adrenaline and put your foot down.

But you can't nebulise a mental-health crisis. You can't inject an episode of depression with a shot of happiness like you can a diabetic hypo with glucagon. In this arena, things are not so quantifiable, so linear.

When I started in the job, I'd get tongue-tied on jobs like this. There was no script to act out, no set strategy to follow; there were no guidelines that told you how to interact. I felt as if I was constantly improvising in an attempt to do the right thing – especially when patients were in an indeterminate state and their problems involved more than just their psychiatric health – family issues, addictions, lack of employment or routine, complex social situations. There were signs to look out for, and mistakes to avoid; there were certain questions you needed to show you had asked in case something went wrong. But that was little help in terms of the ebb and flow of a real-life encounter: people aren't surveys to be crossed off like a multiple choice.

Physical emergencies involved specific problems with targeted treatments; as long as you could identify the cause you could give the appropriate response. But on the mental-health calls, and the social and relational crises that got categorised as such, I wasn't treating a generic illness; I was attempting to engage with a complex and often disordered individual, to establish, in the midst of their problem, what could or should be done. This was less about responding as a clinician, and more about being the closest human being to hand, someone who was willing to listen and who wasn't involved. There was no pocket book for this stuff.

My initial reaction had been a sense that it was our responsibility to solve every problem we came across – because we were the ones who'd been called, and were often the last resort. But with time I realised this was not always within our power, or remit – or even what the patient required. Encounters with patients like James taught me to use a different part of my skill-set, a different part of my personality perhaps. I can't just hand him a medicine, and I can't magic away his long-term problems. What I can do is engage with him as a human being – and try to keep him safe. In the end, patients like James actually require a more genuine response, a more nuanced human interaction, than the glamorous, traumatic emergency calls that take all the plaudits in the 999 CV.

James. I get it that you don't want to go. But I don't really want to leave you here like this. And I'm worried about that arm. Some of those cuts are deep.

I know what I'm doing. I can keep it clean, change the dressings, all of that.

It won't heal properly.

Have you seen the rest of my arms?

He points at the scores of tallied scratches up both forearms. He's obviously right-handed: those on his left arm are much neater. He says he knows what he's doing, he's done it so many times. He doesn't even see it as dangerous any more.

But you know it could be.

I've been told all the stories. Infections. Bleeding. All of that. But I'm still here, aren't I? Look, I know it's fucked up to do this to yourself. I'm not pretending, I'm not an idiot. But so are a lot of things that people do.

Do you have a plan to hurt yourself again?

Not now. You worried? You can take that razor away if you want.

You don't have any others?

No.

Okay. Do you feel any better?

You mean since I cut myself?

That's not exactly what I meant.

I feel different. Better? I don't know.

Does it hurt?

Now?

Yeah.

He thinks.

It hurts. But I knew it was going to.

You knew it was going to hurt?

I knew what it was gonna feel like.

James, I have to ask. Are you thinking of doing anything else?

You worried I'm gonna top myself? You worried you'll get the blame?

Not exactly.

But there's a hint of a smile now. James has had this conversation many times before. He's had plenty of encounters with ambulance and police in the past, and he knows the position we're in.

We can't solve his problems. So what can we do to help? Make him feel slightly less alone in the world, even for a short time. We don't have the training of the psychiatric liaisons, or their access to services, but this is really just a question of humanity: maybe that's all he wants.

We try to persuade him to come to hospital, but he refuses and there's no grounds to force him. I look for reassurances he's not a serious risk to himself. I fill in the requisite form, the one that has little to do with helping him, but will look good when my paperwork is evaluated in an office in three months' time. I refer him to an out-of-hours doctor, for what it's worth.

On the way out, we notice the friendly poster by the front door again and, unsure if we're doing the right thing, we make sure we close the door behind us.

241

XXIII

A 999 call is rarely what it seems. It makes bold claims, but there's always a detail you don't get told. Some hidden context or family drama, a miscommunication or a panicked mix-up: something that colours the simple facts. Medical crises never happen in a vacuum, and one of the first things I learnt in this job is that things are rarely as bad as they sound.

And, just occasionally, they're worse.

55-YR-OLD MALE. NEAR FAINT, IN A PARK

This has been triaged in no-man's-land. It's given as a near faint but the job states the patient's conscious. The resulting priority is *'Category 2, No Back-Up'*: serious enough to trigger an eight-minute response, with a car dispatched on blue lights; not serious enough to warrant a vehicle that can transport the patient to hospital – I will have to ask for one when I get on scene. This is the dispatch equivalent of bagging up your dog waste but then leaving the little black sack on the pavement instead of carrying it to a bin.

The patient could be 'big sick'. Maybe a drop in blood pressure has made him faint. Maybe his heart's developed a strange rhythm. He might have low blood sugar. It could be a heart attack, a blood clot, a stroke. He could be having a snooze. Or he could be drunk. With the age of the patient and the vagueness of the call, anything is possible, and he's in a public place so that may be a complicating factor.

I pull up and I'm waved towards a football pitch a hundred yards away. My risk antenna registers a tiny upgrade. Three men in sports gear are knelt around a figure lying on the wet grass. The word *cardiac* pops into my brain. I grab my bags and the defib and head towards the group.

As I approach, the clues assemble in my brain. Nothing hazardous jumping out. The patient is breathing but his eyes are closed. His body has tone; he's holding up his head. No signs of booze. No blood. No vomit. No weapons. He's still on the ground even though it's wet; they haven't moved him to the nearby bench – why not? The bystanders are concerned but calm: no signs of panic or an argument or a fight. The patient's clothes are sporty but loose: he's been exercising but only casually. His face and hair and clothes are wet; it was raining earlier but this is not from the rain.

But the most telling sign is the patient's colour. His skin is grey. Not white or pink or pale peach like a 1980s bathroom suite. Grey. Grey like slush on a dirty pavement. Grey like smoke from a sugar-beet plant. Grey like a tombstone.

By the time I've reached the patient's side, before I've found out what's happened – before I know the patient's name – I'm convinced there's something wrong with this man's heart.

And if I had time to think about it, I'd admit that the thought gives me a little vocational thrill.

I get the story from one of the friends. *His name's Neil.* Feel the pulse at the wrist. *A kick-about in the park, nothing strenuous.* Pulse a little slow; sats probe on. *Started feeling dizzy.* Blood pressure cuff. Can't reach the upper arm. *Went very pale.* Cut the sleeve. *Helped him to the ground.* Pulse is slow, oxygen's okay. *Hasn't mentioned any pain. But not said a lot.* BP's low. Right-sided heart attack? Grab the ECG leads and dots. *Hasn't passed out but seems confused – not quite with it.* Press in on the radio: time to upgrade. *Bit of heart trouble. High blood pressure? Angina we think.* Stick on the ECG dots. The sweat, the grass: everything's wet; they keep falling off. *Some tests last week. An angiogram?* Holding the leads in place on the chest, the ECG starts to print. The radio buzzes.

Red base. My current assigned. Can you make this a Hot 1? (Critical assistance required.)

There are days when I feel like I'm playing catch-up. One step behind. An expert at arriving once the excitement's done. Patients who were fitting have stopped; those who had fainted have come round and caught the bus home. The baby who'd gone blue and lifeless is now bawling and bright red. The man who was screaming with pain is snoring away.

Several times I'm in the right place at the right time and arrive in a matter of moments. I'm greeted with a wide-eyed *'Wow! You were so quick!'*, as if I've turned up early for a party and they've not quite finished blowing up the balloons. Should I go away and come back later?

There are other days when I get to a job before the problem has even occurred. These are the calls that are made in advance: people who feel like they're about to faint, or are convinced they're going to have a fit. There's the call for a man who looks like he's about to fall over, and the man who's worried he's going to get chicken pox in a few days because his partner's just had it and he's not sure what to do. There are even times when I've been pre-booked – to a bus station for a patient unconscious on a bus that's still ten minutes away.

And then, every once in a while, I arrive at a patient just as their world is about to cave in.

The man in front of me is going to arrest. Collapse. Stop breathing. Of this I'm sure. He's becoming less responsive; his body is going into standby. His heart is undergoing some kind of cataclysm – electrical and vascular – and is threatening to throw in the towel. It will stop beating effectively and will stop pumping blood to the brain.

If he's lucky, his heart will adopt an arrhythmia that it can be shocked out of: patients who go into ventricular fibrillation in the presence of ambulance crews have good survival rates. But in my experience this tends to be a sudden change rather than a gradual deterioration, and this patient's giving off every warning sign in the book.

The heart trace has printed out. It's a very shaky reading: sweaty patients on wet grass are a challenge for a machine that reads tiny electrical signals. But the message is clear – the shape of the trace is ugly and morose: it suggests there's a blockage in the coronary arteries which is causing an arrhythmia and a reduced pumping action. All of which might be workable if the patient didn't already look like death.

What I'm witnessing – participating in – is the drastic descent of a man towards his demise. Within half an hour, he has gone from kicking a ball about with his friends to languishing in the Grim Reaper's departure lounge. The big question is whether the descent can be stopped. What I do in the next ten minutes might not make any difference at all – but it might determine if the patient lives or dies.

There are appropriate civilised responses to this situation – compassion, empathy, hand-wringing and so on – but these would be of little help now. What I feel instead is the exhilaration of a utensil being put to proper use – a long way from the hesitancy of my early days. The moment falls into the rhythm of my processing – a rare convergence of training, practice and circumstance – and there's a guilty elation at being the one who's in the thick of it. My own pulse accelerates; the brain works that little bit faster. I anticipate and respond. Anything surplus gets put aside. Now I'm not so much triaging the patient as triaging my own actions. What can I do for this patient, and in which order does it need to be done?

I plug in an oxygen mask and strap it to the patient's face. I talk to the patient, explaining what I'm doing, but he's barely speaking now. I send one of the bystanders to my car for some extra drugs and equipment, and another to flag down the ambulance crew. I abandon the ECG leads and put defib pads on the patient's chest. I grab my cannula roll and look for a vein in the patient's arm: not much on offer but I make an attempt and seem to have access. Every few seconds I glance at the defib screen to check the rhythm and keep an eye on the blood pressure and pulse, and listen out for the sirens of the ambulance backing me up.

Has he got family?

His wife's on the way.

In my head I run through the drugs I could give, but the situation is changing all the time. The patient still has a pulse but now his breathing's slowing down, becoming heavy. I grab the bag-valve mask, put the patient on his back. The ambulance has pulled up. I grip the patient's chin to the mask and gently squeeze oxygen from the bag. Quick glance at the screen: a slow rhythm, but still compatible with life. I hope the crew can see what's developing. I glance across the field at them. Relief: it's a crew I know and they're on-the-ball; I'll have less to explain.

I tell them what's happened as we slide the patient onto a yellow carry sheet: a tough rectangle with handles up the sides. It's clear to all of us we're on the threshold of a full resus. The patient's friends look shocked, but they help carry him to the edge of the park. It's an awkward business, with lots of equipment attached, but it's simplified by the vigour of necessity.

As we place him on the trolley bed, I realise that at some point in the last two minutes the patient has stopped being Neil, a man I was treating in the park, and has become a body, a broken machine we're doing things to in an attempt to get it working again. This reconfiguration is a seamless, involuntary process; a protective mechanism perhaps, or a path to greater efficiency of thought when faced with what is, in the end, a physical problem. Is this the fate of all my patients now – to become anonymous hosts of puzzles for me to solve?

It's at this moment that the patient goes into cardiac arrest.

He no longer has a carotid pulse, so his brain is not receiving fresh, oxygenated blood; nor are his other major organs. If his body is making any effort to breathe, it's negligible. Without a circulating blood supply, the life-sustaining processes will begin to shut down.

The heart monitor shows there's still activity in his heart: the electrical pathways are still attempting to activate the cardiac muscle in the correct sequence, and the muscle itself may be contracting, but it's too weak to do its job.

This is not what I had hoped for.

I want to look at the screen and see ventricular fibrillation (VF). This will improve the patient's chances. Heart attacks frequently induce VF; this is what happened with Samuel. Because this disordered rhythm occurs abruptly and can often be corrected with a targeted shock, patients who are otherwise healthy but have suffered a cardiac event can sometimes make remarkably good recoveries – especially if they arrest in public or, even better, in an ambulance. Patients who have endured an episode of VF, if quickly reversed, have been known to ask if they've just had a little sleep; there are even tales of them finishing the sentences they had started beforehand.

Unfortunately, disastrously, this patient's heart has bypassed VF and subsided into something called pulseless electrical activity, or PEA. The electrics are working but the plumbing's kaput.

And, as the patient's wife arrives and asks what's going on, I'm beginning to sense this patient will not be coming back.

I'm afraid it looks like Neil's had a heart attack. I have to be completely honest with you, and I'm sorry to be so blunt. He's not breathing, and his heart's not beating for itself. We're doing those things for him.

The words sound redundant – she can see Neil's world is collapsing – but they still need to be said. She hugs her elbows to her chest and holds her hands across her face.

We set up the resuscitation on the trolley in the car park. We send blood around his body by pushing on his chest. We insert an airway and squeeze oxygen into his lungs with the bag. We give the appropriate drugs. It takes a few minutes to get everything running methodically, but these are the golden moments: if we're to make a difference, it will be now.

We get no response.

We load the patient onto the ambulance, alert the hospital and set off on blue lights. All the way there, we keep pushing on the chest, squeezing air into the lungs, pushing drugs into the veins. But the electrical signals are dying out.

By the time we reach the hospital, the patient's heart has lost any sign of spontaneous activity. We hand him over to the hospital team. They continue the treatment for a short while, pushing, squeezing, just as we've done.

And then they stop.

XXIV

It's a bright and merciless autumn day: the kind you have to
lean into to make any progress; a day to leave your umbrella
at home. We park in a wind tunnel behind the FRU. The
tower block's entry panel is smashed, but the communal door
is unlocked anyway. There are sacks in the lobby and a puddle
in the lift, and the mirror is smeared with what's hopefully
ketchup. Something in here stinks. We rattle skywards under
a flickering light and step out into the corridor. We knock
at the flat and wait. Eventually, a woman in a dressing gown
opens the door and stares at our feet. She is hunched and
jowly, with thinning hair and pale, puffy flesh.

Morning, madam.

She doesn't answer.

Did you call the ambulance?

She watches the floor.

Is our colleague here?

She says nothing, but stands aside to let us into the gloom.

Hello . . .? Anyone there?

In here!

We follow the voice to a narrow bedroom down the hall. It contains a single bed, a chest of drawers and two human beings. The first responder is bent double with her back to us. She is stretching across something below: the second human being, a sprawling assembly of folded limbs and greasy flesh that looks like it's been rolled up and dumped unceremoniously on the floor, half under the bed. I can see a foot, an arm and two substantial buttocks, extravagantly hairy and partially covered with a pair of shorts: the rest is unidentifiable meat. A vision of a disastrous game of Twister flashes through my mind.

The position is a mystery, but the real concern is the sound escaping from the patient's throat. Each time he takes a breath, as the sweat-slick skin is stretched and squeezed, a sordid pharyngeal grunt, more painful than a groan, more sinister than a snore, is dragged out of his shuddering bulk and dispatched into the cramped obscurity of the room:

Phnnng-Grouyikkkk!

Then the tiny whistles and clicks of a machine in freefall, until the toil of another great gasp is renewed:

Phnnng-GROUYIKKKKKKKK!

These are the sounds of someone who knows nothing about what's going on; the sounds of something about to fall apart.

This used to be a job for life. The whims of industry would rise and fall, and careers would come and go, but the one thing you could rely on is that people would always get sick. You'd never run out of customers in this trade.

You'd join as a technician, maybe after a few years on patient transport or in care work or the forces. You'd do your time on the road, then work towards your bag and become a medic. If you got a decent crewmate, someone you could trust and tolerate for twelve hours straight, like an alternative spouse in a bizarre arranged marriage, you were set for the long haul. If you were ambitious, you applied for placements on the helicopter or critical care. If you were sick of the patients or injured, you did a secondment with resources or complaints. If you were lazy, so the joke went, you moved into management. And if you were unsociable, like me, you went on the car.

Something has changed along the way. People come and learn the ropes, and you turn around and they're gone. Turnover of road staff has risen, and very few stay with the job long-term.

Maybe this is ambition. People used to arrive with a bit of history and some gratitude for a new endeavour. I was one of them. Nowadays it's all uni graduates and *where am I going next?* Most paramedics appear as fully formed clinicians in their early twenties with grand plans, dealing with the banalities of death before they've learnt how to bleed a radiator or season a Bolognese. There's less of a sense of a career that's a destination, a pinnacle, more of it being a stepping stone along the way. Or perhaps they're trying to escape?

I often hear about the alternatives available to paramedics: to work in A&E departments or doctors' surgeries; as urgent-care practitioners, community educators. Yet most of these opportunities involve turning your back on the invigorating chaos of pre-hospital care for something more sedate. Perhaps this is just about clinical progression, but I suspect there's something less positive going on. It's as if there's a new atmosphere these days – a growing sense that, if you're not careful, this job will get you in the end.

Like a green flamingo, our colleague has stretched awkwardly across the patient to put on oxygen, attach ECG leads, check everything measurable that could have brought this colossus to the floor. All the numbers look normal. There's no sign of a head injury or a seizure or low blood sugar. Even his oxygen levels, in spite of that pained inhalation, look good. So why is he tangled up in an unresponsive heap in the corner of this tiny darkened room?

The arrangement looks calculated for awkwardness. It's as if someone has dragged his defenceless frame here and knotted it up in an act of malice. He must surely be in considerable pain – if his body is even registering pain. There's also the constrictive element: face down, backside up, disordered and restrained, it's little surprise he's working so hard on the basics.

We can move him to make him more comfortable, but the real question is why he's like this in the first place. Did he fall, or faint, or crawl, or hide? Was he looking for something? Did his brain, in a moment of deranged sabotage, cause him to assume a pose of maximum impediment? We can only guess. He is a machine with faulty wiring. A defeated trophy and the snare it's caught in. An escapologist who's forgotten how to break out.

He can tell us nothing, cannot respond even to basic

commands. We ask the woman who let us in – perhaps his mother? – for help:

Excuse me, madam. Can you tell us what happened?

But she mutters and hides her face and walks away.

Will you talk to us, please? Is this man your son?

She ducks into the bathroom –

Madam?

– and locks the door. She must have called the ambulance, but she hasn't spoken since we arrived.

Our working assumption is that there's been a sudden disruption of his brain function, but we can only guess how, and we're not going to find out much more here. He needs blood tests, a scan, A&E. We're unlikely to fix anything now – or make him any easier to move.

What we're left with, then, is less a clinical problem than a logistical challenge. We need to get him off the floor, onto a chair, out to the ambulance, into hospital. This is our basic function in the world. We request a second crew, but we're not going to stand around watching him deteriorate while we wait.

He's an expanded dead weight: a slippery conglomeration of flaccid, flabby flesh. He has no tone to push or pull against, no handles to latch onto. Every angle is overlaid with corpulence; every edge is sculpted like wet clay. He is pure, stubborn gravity.

Getting sick people from their private predicament to a hospital bed is a fundamental – perhaps *the* fundamental – of ambulance work. But at what cost? The very traits that render patients immobile – size, weakness, physical degeneration – are the traits that put such a strain on the people charged with their care.

Advances in lifting equipment have filtered through to ambulance work. In the out-of-hospital setting, however, where houses are cluttered and people find the most ingenious places to collapse – hugging the toilet, up a tree, against an inward-opening door, half-in and half-out of a loft hatch – equipment is only part of the answer, no matter how smart the engineering. So, when time is of the essence, moving a cumbersome, uncooperative body out of a tight spot often comes down to quick thinking, improvisation – and brute force.

There's a perception that this is an energetic profession: out and about, lifting and carrying, mostly on your feet. But in fact it's pretty sedentary. We may be away from a desk, but we still spend a lot of time on our backsides. The physical elements are sporadic enough to lack much benefit and, like the problem facing us today, sudden and singular enough to increase the chance of injury. Any notion of this career being a way of staying in shape is a myth belied by the extent of the collective sick-note.

It's the shoulders from lifting. It's the knees from bending, or kneeling to do CPR. It's the twinges you thought were things of the past. The reaching awkwardly, the uncooperative loads. Old sports injuries making a reappearance after a long week of shifts. And of course, our backs.

None of this is exceptional, but there are other factors taking their toll. For many it's the years of rotating shifts: a kind of permanent jetlag making its presence felt in the fuzzy head or the confused bowels or the racing heart or the darkened mind. Some bodies seem to run out of steam, or never recover beyond a certain point. People go off long-term sick, and never return. Personalities lurch in unexpected directions – maybe knocked off course by what they've seen, or the lurking spectre of vicarious grief. Sometimes resentment curdles, or bitterness arrives; perhaps an addiction begins to pull at the seams or a relationship breaks down and the work is suddenly too close to the bone. Though we might not want to admit it, in the end we're just like the patients whose struggles we glimpse in tiny fractions each day.

For some, in work terms, these problems are the final straw; for others they might be the beginning of the end. For all of us, in a career where we're still expected to carry patients down the stairs until we're sixty-seven, at the very least these are persistent warnings that the future might need to adapt its plans.

Our anonymous, moribund patient has one thing in his favour: he's collapsed on a laminate floor. By moving furniture and clutching a bodily protrusion each, we are able to slide him, one haul at a time, backwards out of the bedroom and into the relative clearing of the living room, tucking a sheet underneath to stop the wet skin sticking to the glossy flooring, and barging the sofa out of the way until he comes to rest, flopped on his side like a giant newborn. His body has shown no reaction to this onslaught, but unfolded, released, it relaxes and his breathing becomes calmer, quieter, more familiar.

Now he's in the open we can see his face. He becomes an individual.

Sir? Can you hear us, sir? Can you open your eyes?

We still don't know his name.

We've moved you from the bedroom. Okay? Now we need to get you onto our chair. We're going to take you to hospital. Can you squeeze my hand?

Like an Easter Island *moai*, everything about him is over-sized and top-heavy: his balding head a glossy dome, his square jaw an outcrop, his bloated face a mask embellished with hairy ears and a flattened nose. We shine a light in his eyes: the pupils react but he does not turn away. How much of this is new? How long was he down? Along one cheek a trampled cherry of flesh bears the imprint of the bedroom floor, and his beard and moustache are slathered with saliva and snot. We wipe his face, and the sweat from his head.

Our next challenge is to get this dead weight from the floor to the chair. Lifting, we realise, is not an option: every time we strain to heave him upwards, he slips from our hands, and the centre of gravity never leaves the floor. We turn him on his side and fold him at right angles at hip and knee, then lie the carry chair on its side on the floor and slide it into place behind him, so that his body shape is fitted to the chair's configuration. We strap him on using the seatbelts, then roll the chair, and the patient with it, onto its back, to put the patient into a horizontal sitting position. We then anchor the back wheels and tip the chair forwards to an upright position. None of this is elegant or easy, but it works. We wrap a blanket around him, tighten the straps, secure the oxygen again, scan the flat for any information, and make our way to the soggy lift.

As we wheel the patient to the truck, a cloud of dust whips into our faces, and a blue plastic bag wraps itself around my leg. The local pigeons are hurled sideways, dodging balconies and satellite dishes, and lines of trees bow in unison, paying their respects.

In the ambulance we use the blanket to drag him from the chair, straining our sinews in awkward postures, and with one final lurch we deposit him on the bed – about half a minute before the second crew arrive to help.

Oh. You seem to have things under control?

Yep. Good timing, guys . . .

We let the hospital know we're coming, and set off.

We'll hand the patient over to a casual doctor and never find out what caused his curious plunge or what happened to him as a result: just another silent soul who's been our focus for an hour and then vanished for ever. Tomorrow we'll feel the twinges in our backs.

Someone asked me recently if this job has a shelf-life. It's a pertinent phrase: the idea that you can do this kind of thing only for so long. If working on an ambulance is the job it's intended to be – essential, fulfilling, varied, secure – then surely there shouldn't be a limit as to how much of it you can take? As I was about to find out, this was not always the case.

XXV

The boyfriend greets us with the immortal phrase:

She doesn't know you're coming.

I've heard these words before, and they never lead to anything good. Then he says:

I don't think she'll be very happy when she sees you.

This is not what we want to be told.

Okay. Do you want to let her know we're here?

He hasn't told her because he knows she'll be mad. That means there's a world of trouble going on. He's delayed the confrontation, hoping our uniforms will water it down, but this rarely works: now she'll feel conspired against as well.

When we follow him in, she turns her head. Her eyes have the hooded wrath of inebriation:

Who the fuck. Are they. And why. The fuck. Are they here?

She's perched on a sofa, holding a rucksack on her lap.

Take it easy, baby.

He walks across to touch her shoulder, but she stands and roars him away –

Get! Off me!

– then fall-sits back down. He spreads his hands:

Okay. Chill. I just called them to help you.

She slams her fist on the coffee table.

I don't need any fuckin' help!

She lifts her eyes to take us both in. Her movements are lurching; her words stilted:

I don't wanna be touched. I've been. Through this before. I know my rights, officers.

They're not the police, Jas.

Shut up! I'm telling you. Now. I don't wanna be touched. And if you. If you touch me. That is against my wishes and that. That is an assault. So don't. Fuckin' touch me, okay?

I'm not sure what we've walked into. There's the echo of a lover's tiff, but also something more menacing. There's another woman in the room, trying to mollify the patient, but it's not clear if she's family, a friend, a housemate, or some component of the problem.

When the job was dispatched, it mentioned an overdose. My guess is the boyfriend's done something to upset Jas, and that's opened a floodgate to some bigger problems. Now he wants us to wave a magic wand. The patient doesn't even want us here. I think she's dealt with the emergency services before and I have my suspicions where this is heading. I look to the boyfriend:

What's going on?

Restless and resistant, Jas stands and starts stalking the room, nearly tripping on the low table. The boyfriend tells us about some tablets, some alcohol, but she cuts him off with an elaborate stagger and a swing of her bag. She approaches us and fairly spits out her words:

Mind. Your.

then comes right up to my face

Fuckinnnn'. Business.

and stomps out of the flat. The second woman, whoever she is, scurries after her.

Minding my business would be fine with me. But I'm pretty sure that's not where things are headed tonight.

My main concern is our location. The flat's on the first floor. The front door opens onto an external landing that runs along the front of the building, linking each of the flats to the stairwell, the drop shielded by nothing more than a waist-high balustrade. We follow along the balcony to the stairs. She's gone up to the second floor.

It's unclear what's happened, and we don't have time to find out. We know Jas is upset and aggressive, probably drunk. Something in her demeanour suggests a history of extreme behaviours. I suspect she's capable of doing something quite dangerous – to herself or someone else.

We climb the stairs and find her sat against the wall, shouting abuses down the steps. I tell her my name and ask if I can talk to her about what's been going on.

No you fuckin' can't.

I've already pressed in on my radio and now it buzzes. I step away for a moment:

Red base, can you please dispatch the police on our current assigned?

Roger that. Are you safe?

We're safe, but the patient's upset and aggressive.

Now the boyfriend comes up the stairs. This seems to flick

a switch and suddenly Jas is up on her feet and kicking the railings, pulling at the handrail, stretching towards him and firing out a stream of vitriol that rises in volume and pitch until it splits into a scream. Her frantic accusations become more specific, more obscene, interspersed with claims of violence done to her, boasts of wounds she has inflicted on him, threats that she will do the same again. I don't like where this is going, and I want to take the heat out of the room. I step towards her:

Jas, please. Look at me for a second.

She stops and stares at me, wild-eyed and full of hate:

Don't. Fuckin'. Come near me.

Suddenly her unsteadiness is a thing of the past. She is abruptly sober: poised, primed, ready to pounce. I turn to the boyfriend:

Mate, do you want to go back downstairs? Give her a moment?

I don't need a fuckin' moment!

But he's more than happy to grab a bit of space. As he goes, she leans over the railing and rains curses and spittle down on his head. He stops and responds with an accusation of his own – something about a night she spent with his friend. This does not calm her down.

With him out of sight, she paces the tiny landing, looking for a new target. She grabs her rucksack from the floor, swings back the door and walks out onto the communal balcony. A lump of dread rises in my throat. She approaches the railing and dangles her bag over the barrier, then drops it. After a moment it hits the ground below with a smash.

Come away from there, Jas.

But she doesn't come away. She takes hold of the horizontal bar with each hand and lifts her right foot up. She has heavy laced boots and tight jeans and a combat-type jacket. Her foot rests on the top of the handrail, then she puts it forward and stretches her leg over the edge and hooks her knee on the bar.

No, no, don't do that.

I say this as much to myself as to her.

She hoists herself up and leans to her left and rolls her torso and her backside so that she's straddling the bar, about seven, maybe eight metres above the concrete, and at this point she's at least halfway over the rail, and showing no sign of turning back.

This is happening. Something needs to be done.

I'm thinking a bunch of things and they're all there at once. Does she really want to jump? Am I willing to find out? Will a two-storey drop kill her? That depends how she lands. It's high enough to cause some serious harm. Does not touching include stopping her from breaking her leg, or worse? And finally, selfishly, soberly: if she jumps and I'm stood right beside her, just how bad will it look?

These thoughts are the work of a moment, but they're elbowed aside by a more instinctive response.

I reach out and grab the loose material of her jacket. I get a good handful and pull it back towards me. My feet spread themselves into a wide stance, and I take a step back as I pull: I don't want to follow if she's determined to fall. There's a moment when it could go either way, but then, with a swift heave, she tips back towards me and her legs roll round and her feet drop down onto the balcony and she lands upright on the right side of the bar.

There's something in the smoothness of the motion and the fact she doesn't immediately try again that makes me wonder if she really meant it, but I'll never know. She was certainly close enough. Within a moment her boyfriend is out on the balcony and together we manoeuvre her back inside.

I press in on my radio again, to update Control and find out about the police. I'd like them here sooner rather than later. Jas has allowed herself to be steered away from the edge, but she's still shouting and screaming. She's not about to break down in remorseful cooperation. This struggle is far from over.

I stand in front of the door back out to the balcony, shutting us all into this strange, brick cavern at the top of the stairs. If she decides to go back out there, I will block her way.

This is exactly what happens, about two minutes later. Having flirted with composure, she's once again enraged by something – it's no longer clear what – and makes an abrupt grab for the door. My feet are up against its frame and it doesn't budge. She yanks at the metal handle, once –

Move!

– twice –

Let me out!

– three times –

Bastard!

– shouting in violent punctuation, just as I spot the police car pulling up a hundred yards down the road. Then my radio buzzes with a response. I lift it to my chin just as Jas, having failed to force the door open, makes a more direct attack.

She reaches up and grabs me with her left hand, while trying to pull the door with her right.

Get out of my way, you bastard!

Her left arm extends round the back of my neck and she stretches her thumb and fingers as far to each side as she can get them, clamping my neck muscles in a kind of Vulcan grip.

Let me out!

Her nails burrow into the flesh on either side, and she squeezes with the febrile vigour of a creature with nothing to lose.

All clinicians are familiar with duty of care. I had it drilled into me from day one. This commitment – to take responsibility, in a spirit of diligence and professionalism, for another person's welfare – seems so basic an impulse, so fundamental a notion, it hardly needs to be taught. How could such an essential project be derailed? What could possibly stop a carer from caring?

Consider a patient who doesn't want to be helped. The clinician wants to do their duty, but the patient won't let them. They might indicate their reluctance with a polite verbal refusal – or they might demonstrate it by committing an assault.

In most professional encounters, a physical attack would signal the end of the interaction. If you attacked an opponent (or, worse, an official) in a sporting contest, you probably wouldn't finish the match. Staff in all professions have a right, we're frequently told, to work in an environment free from harm or abuse. Real life, of course, is rarely that simple.

If a clinician were to approach an intoxicated patient and then get punched, they might reasonably retreat and leave the patient to their own devices. But what if the intoxication caused the patient to walk towards a busy road or a train line? Should the clinician accept their injury as a kind of battle scar, and go back for more in order to prevent a greater harm? Given the volatility of the patient, is it fair or even safe to expect them to intervene again?

We might assume that a patient who's violent because their faculties are impaired is still vulnerable. The duty of care, therefore, endures. But, in an ideal world, that duty should only be discharged in the presence of protection for the carers. After all, the road or train line also poses a risk to them.

The reality in this job is that when most of these dilemmas arise, such protection is yet to arrive. The fluctuating dynamics of the real world rarely match up with the strait-laced hypotheticals of an imagined scenario.

In my experience, hostile behaviours arise from different causes. Patients can be aggressive due to illness: an agitated diabetic having an episode of low blood sugar; a delirious pensioner with a nasty urine infection. In these cases, a lack of oxygen or glucose inhibits the functioning of the brain.

There are also patients who present a different challenge, because there's something psychotic going on: a perceptive disconnection which causes them to transgress the accepted boundaries of behaviour. And then there are those who experience interactive disturbances after taking chemical substances which alter their psychological processing.

Physical and neurological problems such as these can be treated or managed – some more easily than others. Usually, once the underlying cause is remedied, behaviours calm down. But, of course, there are also those patients whose hostility has no easily correctable physiological cause.

Red base, can you update the police, we need them in the stairwell on the second floor?

Her vice-hand is still clamped to the back of my neck.

Can you tell them the patient tried to jump from the balcony? And now she's attacking us . . .

She's grabbing at the door, trying to prise me away so she can get out, and squeezing with all her might. What's odd, in hindsight, is that I don't just strike back. In the heat of the moment, you'd expect yourself to retaliate, to do enough to make your assailant stop: push her away, swing an arm, knock her legs, do something worse. But I'm also trying to hold that door closed, and instead I utter the rather polite words:

Stop that, please.

And when this command lacks the desired effect, I say:

Get your hands off my neck.

But she doesn't.

My colleague comes to intercede –

Let go, let go!

– and the boyfriend grabs at her arm, but she's like a slippery eel, squirming this way and that, relentless, aberrant, offloading her anger in a wide-eyed spasm. I hold fast to the door and twist away and duck my head, and eventually her claws are prised away.

Untethered, off-balance, she spins about the tiny landing. We watch to see what she'll do next. There's a sense that all the shackles are off. Feeling the numbers, the shock perhaps, she reels away towards the stairs and, yelling still, she step-stumbles down the first few steps. An opportunity.

Okay, let's keep moving, let's get downstairs.

We usher her on, coaxing, guiding, muttering instructions with forced placidity, a motley ring of figures lolloping towards a solution, surrounding her at arm's length, watching closely for another outburst. She stops and turns, shouts some more, but her rage has passed over the summit and, like her body on the stairs, begun a kind of weary descent. I go ahead for the last few steps, and as I open the communal door to let the officers in, things have suddenly become surprisingly calm.

I don't know if you've ever watched the children of a close friend trash your house for you? Paragliding off furniture, playing rugby with family heirlooms, checking the tensile strength of your prized possessions – that sort of thing? The whole experience can become rather uncomfortable – especially when the parents sit there with you, and do nothing to intervene.

Initially, as a generous host, you give them a bit of leeway, assuming your friends are employing a progressive form of parenting, and will soon step in. But gradually, as time goes on, and your possessions take a more permanent battering, you begin to realise that they're going to do no such thing.

You're faced with a dilemma. You don't want to be a kill-joy, but you feel pretty strongly that a line needs to be drawn in the sand. And while the sand may be yours, the responsibility for drawing that line lies squarely with your friends. You feel a bit of discipline is the order of the day. Maybe a punishment. At least a stern word. It never comes.

So as the peptic anger burns inside your chest, you start to feel rather undermined. Something significant and improper has occurred, and you're expecting a proportionate response from the authorities, or at least some kind of acknowledgement. What you're offered, instead, is the sight of the parents humouring their children in an attempt to avoid a scene. Just as one of your treasured LPs is frisbeed across the living room, and no word of rebuke is forthcoming, you begin to wonder if maybe it's you who has the problem – perhaps you're wrong to feel this sense of inequity?

When we open the door and inform the officers that the patient has tried to jump from the second-floor balcony, and that we've physically prevented her from doing so, and that she's subsequently assaulted one of us, and is still exhibiting signs of anger and violence now, they do not immediately clap on a pair of handcuffs and read Jas her rights. They do not put her under a Section 136, detaining her in a public place for threatening harm to self or others. They don't call for the van and back-up. They don't even look very cross.

What they do instead is begin chatting to the patient as if they're attempting to win her trust: making tentative forays to determine the lie of the land, like a builder stepping onto a dubious-looking flat roof.

These are ambulance tactics. We're the ones who put in a charm offensive with difficult individuals – because that's the only thing we can do. But, in my mind at least, we've got beyond that stage and something a bit more severe is required.

As I walk away for a moment, waiting for the adrenaline tremors to wear off, I start to wonder if I've got this wrong. Perhaps I'm the one at fault? I'd expected to see my rights being asserted in some way; I'd expected some show of authority. Instead I'm faced with the spectacle of an unrepentant individual being cajoled, indulged, by the people we had called to assist us. The message is clear: they're here in case things get feisty again, a physical presence, a visible warning sign, a bit of chat. The rest is up to us.

The result is a surreal hour spent outside the property, trying to persuade a patient who's just assaulted me to come to hospital with me. It's pretty clear we can't leave her here. My neck is red and sore and my hackles are raised and I feel suddenly drained. This job is thankless. I know now why I didn't react to try to stop her – because I saw this coming; in retrospect, any sense of protection has done exactly what I expected it to do – it's disappeared.

I've done my best to be patient, to empathise, to intervene. I've given Jas the benefit of the doubt. Taken her predicament into consideration. Provided her with multiple opportunities to take a different path. She's said and screamed a lot of things, and some of them point to the injuries of her past, and I've borne all this in mind. But tolerance alone can't change any of that; neither can it restrain an aggressor or justify an assault.

At a primal, indignant, wounded level, I'd like nothing better than to leave Jas to it and damn the consequences, because I've had enough. But after everything that's happened, I find myself in the bizarre position of pleading with her to come with us, even while she spits insults into my face, because at one o'clock in the morning it's the only way out of this mess and, ultimately, she's still a patient in our care. It's demeaning and tiresome, and entirely pragmatic.

We can't establish if she has the capacity to make her own choices, because she won't cooperate with our questions or physical checks. At times she seems fully coherent, boasting of the foreign languages she speaks and her superior intellect, reeling off lists of her past accomplishments – which apparently include being prosecuted for assaulting police officers while resisting arrest. I'm not sure if she's trying to impress us, threaten us or encourage us to change careers. She's doing a good job of the latter. But when she's asked a direct question, her only response is to shout racist and homophobic abuse. Plus, of course, we can't ignore the fact she's just tried to jump from a second-floor balcony.

There's a further indulgence as we finally leave scene: we agree to take her to a hospital that's further from here and nearer to her home. It's a simple trade-off to be out of this quagmire. The boyfriend comes with us, and sometimes his presence seems to calm her; at other times he sets her off afresh. At A&E we ask her to be quiet out of respect for the other patients, but this is like asking a cat not to chase a laser:

she makes lurid personal comments about each of the people we pass on the way in.

I tell one of the police officers I want to report the assault, and she takes my details and tells me in the next breath that nothing will come of it:

They'll say she didn't know what she was doing.

She definitely knew what she was doing.

They'll say she was out of control. Not thinking straight.

Okay, but I want it reported, because it still happened.

Of course, of course. But . . . don't expect anything to come of it.

Then, as soon as we get inside the doors, she and her colleague are gone; Jas is someone else's problem now.

Unfortunately, that someone is us, and if I thought the end was in sight, I was wrong. The A&E is bursting at the seams: drunk patients slumped in chairs; a man in a suit reading a novel, oblivious; another group of police waiting with a sullen young man in cuffs; an elderly lady vomiting into a bowl. Jas approaches each of them, bouncing off her boyfriend, who with rolling eyes tries to guide her weakly away. I encourage her to sit, which she does for about a minute. Then she gets restless and stands and begins pacing and the volume rises again. I wonder if tonight will ever be over, as I step towards her and, in as calm a voice as I can muster, ask her if she'll sit down for a minute until we've spoken to the nurse.

Who the fuck are you? Parafuckingmedic! I'm hungry! Get me some food!

Let's tell the nurse what's happened, and find out where they want you. Then we can get you something to eat.

Where's the nearest shop? I want a fuckin' sandwich.

Just wait for a moment.

Don't tell me to fuckin' wait! I want a sandwich. I told you I'm hungry, parafuckingmedic!

By now she's up in my face, leaning her head to the side in that way movie villains do when they want to make something really, really clear.

Do you want me to call security?

This comes from a nurse walking past.

Thank you.

She does. They never materialise.

I'm at the end now, in so many ways. On some naïve, base level, I still find myself wanting the best for Jas – or the version of her that's cowering somewhere underneath this jagged, bitter crust. But I'm stuck with the version of her that seems to delight in casting misery around like so much grain.

I explain to her that she hasn't been detained; she's here voluntarily and free to go to the shop; free to leave if she really wants to. By now I have nothing left to give: I have no powers to make her stay and feel I've done everything I can. Frankly, I'd welcome the peace. But here's the telling thing: in spite of all her rage at being dragged here, 'against my fuckin' will', she doesn't leave. She stays and begins listing, at great length, my personal faults. It's most enlightening.

The small audience of emergency-department tenants watches on, possibly sympathetic, possibly entertained, unquestionably relieved it's not them. After forty minutes of this, the nurse is ready to take a handover. And then a doctor who's been watching from a safe distance asks me:

Does she really need to be here?

And this feels like the bleakest moment of the whole sorry saga. Does he think I'm here for fun?

I'm used to managing volatile patients. Being insulted is routine. Even physical aggression is common enough. What depresses me about tonight's episode – what will hover over me in the coming months and make me wonder why I bother – is not the assault. It's the lack of solidarity or even acknowledgement from the people who, in a different version of the scenario, could easily be the ones on the receiving end. The way the whole episode will disappear into a vacuum of indifference. The sense that all this grasping of the nettle is somehow in vain.

There's a similar response from the official channels. When I report the incident internally, I'm told that nothing can be done because Jas has not given a confirmed address. The investigation concerns itself chiefly with checking if my conflict-resolution training is up to date, subtly shifting the responsibility back to me. And the officer is right about the charges: I never hear a thing. Jas is free to do the same again next time.

For now, I give the nurse a potted description of the last three hours, and let her make up her own mind if Jas really needs to be here. I'm done.

Stepping outside is like that moment when your neighbours turn off the music from an all-night party. That sudden tranquillity. That exhausted, weightless, magical peace. Waiting for the brain-buzz to fade. Shaking the head in disbelief.

We return to station to file an incident report. After a quick tea, but no medals, it's time to go again, because the patients keep calling, and the service never stops, and the next one might be someone who needs our help.

We push the button and go green.

When we return to the hospital a few hours later, we'll find that Jas has been discharged without further care.

XXVI

This is the call no one wants to receive.

Six o'clock, start of shift: we're the first crew to go. Out on the truck, checking equipment, making sure nothing's gone walkabout. Gear loaded, drugs signed out. It's a short shift today and we're hoping for an easy day. As we move around the ambulance, opening cupboards, sipping tea, we talk about what we did yesterday after work: a swim, TV, an early night before another four-thirty alarm. After a long week of early starts, the weekend is approaching. A couple of grannies-down and some walk-on-walk-offs and our work will be done. Time for a decent coffee at some point. Nothing to trouble our brains until at least half-past ten.

There's a knock on the ambulance door and a head appears.

Sorry guys. Control on the phone.

They don't waste any time.

They've sent down a job. Sorry guys, it's an arrest around the corner. It's a paed.

We look at our colleague a moment.

It's not a joke. Sorry. Wish it was.

How old?
Didn't say. Anything you need?
We've got everything, haven't we?
Think so.
He shuts the door.
This is the call no one wants to receive.

The address is a flat on a row of shops. We're there in minutes and so is the car. The door's open because the police are already inside, so we follow along a corridor and down some stairs, into a dark room full of furniture and people: the police, a woman with her hands across her face, an old man in a dressing gown. In the middle of the floor, three officers kneel in a tight group. One is counting, another pushing downwards in time.

Hi, guys, shall we take over?

But they can't hear; their minds are focused on what they're doing. I touch their shoulders.

We're here, guys. Can you let us in?

They turn to see us and their faces flush with relief. These guys deal with tough stuff every day, but this is different. They gladly make way. The one with her hands around the patient's chest asks:

Shall I keep going with compressions?
Please, for the moment.

As they move aside on their knees, the patient is revealed.

A tiny infant in a nappy, flat on its back on the carpeted floor. Pale, floppy, motionless. Perhaps nine months old. Its limbs are splayed outwards. Its torso is a brittle cylinder, carved with ridges, stretched with flesh. Its skin is pink – except that it isn't. Living flesh is a glossy amalgam of flecks and flushes: the cherry glow of perfusion, pencil-blue veins, the metabolic sheen of animated tissue. Tiny discrepancies and variations that speak of life. This child's skin has the flattened, washed-out veneer of the past.

It's a baby with a family, a bed, a cry of its own and no one else's; perhaps a toy or a blanket that helps it sleep. But for now, for the purposes of what we need to do right now, it is simply a human body which is not working and needs to be fixed. A project, a problem, the starting point of an algorithm. There is no context here, no innovation, only process. Seen from the head end, upside down, I don't look at its features, ask its name, even think about whether it's a boy or a girl.

One of my colleagues kneels at the feet and encircles the child's ribcage with her hands, pressing rhythmically in the centre of the chest with her thumbs. Another takes the small bag-valve mask and pulls it into shape, fitting it onto the tiny face to squeeze two cups of oxygen into the pocket-sized lungs. While the compressions are delivered, she slides a tiny airway into the mouth and pushes some padding under the shoulders, to lift the torso slightly and open up the airway. At the next two ventilations, the chest lifts and falls like a regular breath.

A fourth crew member has followed us in. We won't delay on scene, but we want to get things right, want to have a smooth routine in place before moving: once we've corrected what we can, we'll alert the hospital and go.

I apply the defibrillation pads to the doll-like torso: they are industrially sticky on such blameless juvenile skin. The reading appears on the screen: there's no indication of electricity in the child's heart. This is not a surprise. Any flicker of hope is dwindling.

The mother stands off to the side with the police: dazed, sobbing, not looking our way. A second child, perhaps two years old, clambers over the bed right beside where we're resuscitating the baby, unaffected by the influx of strangers, happily watching us attack its sibling as if we're playing some kind of game.

Can someone take this child out of the way?

A police officer lifts the child off the bed and takes it out of the room.

We're told the baby woke once in the night, was comforted and went back to sleep, and when Mum woke up this morning, she found it lifeless in the cot. Mum called a neighbour who called 999. The baby has no medical history and had not been unwell.

We inspect the body for injuries, rashes, bruises, any obvious clues. A quick glance around the room for anything suspicious or concerning. The child's temperature is down but no more than we'd expect; the blood sugar reading is low – not necessarily the cause but something we should correct. Once the fluid line is in place we'll give glucose and adrenaline.

I align the 'EZIO' with the top of the child's shin. It's a small handheld drill with a large needle which will puncture the skin and bore into the bone, so we can give medicines directly into the bloodstream. I squeeze the trigger and the motor whirrs; I advance the needle; the epidermis stretches and pops; the battery fails and then revives; the needle eases into the bone. I remove the needle, leaving the cannula in place, a futuristic port on the surface of the child's skin. It's a piece of torture in the telling, but I don't consider the violence of the act; all I'm thinking is to get it right. All any of us is thinking is to make sure we get this right.

This is a child who has not woken up.

Mum has stirred of her own accord, the first time in months, a dull unease in the back of her throat. As she's gone over to check in the half-light of dawn, no gurgling laugh has greeted her approach, no feet have drummed impatiently on the mattress. Perhaps the child is sleeping still? But when she lifts it from the cot, there's a peculiar heaviness. The child has not wriggled and blinked and buried its head in her shoulder or clutched at her neck. It has not opened its eyes and bounced with excitement. Its face has not lit up. It has remained still. Unresponsive. Inert.

The mother has experienced the horrific plunging moment that every parent dreads. Did she sense the start of her freefall in the silence as she stooped over the cot? Did she know as soon as she saw? Does she even understand now exactly what has happened?

It's time to move. We've done all we can on scene, put everything in its place, taken on our roles, given the best chance we can give in the crucial early moments. We've maximised the provision of oxygen with ventilations and airway management. We've started giving drugs via the fluid line into the bone: small doses of saline, glucose, adrenaline. We've ensured the best quality CPR we can. We've remained as calm and methodical as possible, and put any thoughts of the looming sorrow and the scene of devastation we're working in to one side. We've done nothing more than follow procedure.

The exit to the truck is our next challenge. We need to get up a flight of stairs, along a corridor, out onto the road and up onto the vehicle, all the while keeping the resus going.

It's a three-person operation. I rest the tiny form of the baby along my left forearm, its head in the palm of my hand, its legs either side of my arm. With my other hand I grip the trunk and press rhythmically in the centre of the chest –

One, two, three, four, five, six, seven, eight, nine, ten, eleven, twelve, thirteen, fourteen, fifteen

– while my crewmate supports the head with her hand, holding the airway in place, lifting the chin slightly, and squeezing the bag –

One . . . two . . .

– each time I stop pushing. Our other colleague guides us, while carrying the defib, the oxygen, the attached fluids and drugs.

We move slowly, step by careful step, a lopsided arthropod, two heads forwards, one in reverse, alerting each other to hazards, sidestepping obstacles, counting compressions, eyeing at intervals the rhythm on the screen.

I reverse up the stairs, knocking my heels against the risers to ensure I'm on each step. We reach the top and glide along the corridor —

Two metres to the door frame. There's a little lip and then a step down . . .

— and emerge into the daylight. I wonder if anyone can see us now — will they know what's happened? Will they think of this every time they walk past? Thankfully the streets are quiet — no schoolchildren yet; not many cars. We help each other up into the truck and lay the infant on the bed. It is suddenly tiny again, adrift on a giant white sheet. Nothing here was designed for a child this size. This is not supposed to happen to a creature so small.

I push such thoughts away and focus on the task. It's time to check the rhythm again, give more drugs. We will reposition and reassess and alert the hospital and leave.

Sometimes bad things happen to normal people. We'd rather they didn't, but humans are organisms, not machines. This job exists so that there's someone on hand to answer the call. Crews might grow disillusioned, but it's because bad things happen to normal people that we're here in the first place, and still here now.

That's not to deny the morbid thrill of it all. Blood-soaked trauma and meaty medical conundrums get the brain in gear. Are we sociopaths? I don't think so. Morbidly unhinged? Hopefully not. It's no surprise that crews start to get their kicks from other people's misfortune, because the sicker the patient, the more useful the crew feels; the greater their sense of worth; bluntly, the more interesting their day at work.

As the saying goes, it's not that we want bad things to happen to you; it's just that we want to be there when they do.

But there's one exception. One category of job which any ambulance crew would gladly never go to again: the paediatric cardiac arrest. People in this job can become blasé about pain and violence, and injury and death, but this, without exception, is the call no one wants to receive.

We're on our way to hospital with a child who is not going to survive. We've secured the airway, pushed on the chest, squeezed air into the lungs and given drugs, but we are not going to change the outcome. We know this.

We will continue until we reach the hospital and hand over to the waiting medical team; then we'll retreat to the ambulance and write our paperwork, reorganise our equipment. We've had very little contact with the patient's mother, who has travelled with the police and will be spoken to by the doctors at A&E. We will not have to say to her those definitive words, or explain what has happened and how nothing more could be done. We'll hear her cry from outside, but we won't have to see her face when she is told.

Later, our colleagues will ask if we're okay – because this is the call no one wants to receive. The question feels indulgent: we've not lost our child; what does it matter how we feel? That's the job, isn't it – dealing with tragedy and brokenness and not letting it bring you down? Reaching into the desolation and expecting your hands to come out unscathed?

There's long been a tendency in this job to play down its emotional impact. It's a mutual code of silence, and we all play along. Proudly robust, darkly comic, heroically modest, we're ambulance people and we don't let that kind of thing get to us. When people outside the job ask how we cope, we answer them:

By not thinking about it.

Or:

By it not being you.

Because, no matter how grim, how direct, how involved, the pain belongs to someone else.

I think we've only recently started to admit how unhelpful these attitudes can be. We're more than just remote witnesses; we're involved. And while we might not break down in tears after every nasty job, we need to acknowledge the cumulative effect of rummaging around in the carnage of the world. These things need to be named, acknowledged and given their due. These things affect us; they leave a mark.

Today we have fought a close-up battle for the life of a child, and we've lost. But, taken up with the patient, we've stayed in the present and kept the shattered future away from our minds. This has been a clinical exercise, first and foremost.

For us, this is one job in a week of jobs. A bad job, yes. A memorable, tragic, difficult job. But, ultimately, just a short visit to someone else's heartbreak. We've done our duty, earned our stripes, been through a rite of passage. When we go home, we'll spare a thought for the family whose grief we have witnessed up close. We might talk to our partners, hug our kids extra tight, call a friend. When we close our eyes, we may see the pitiful child's tiny form. The nameless sibling who will never know its sister may clamber off that bed and appear in our dreams. But this was someone else's tragedy, and we'll rip off the Band-Aid and move on. Tomorrow there'll be other jobs, other patients. The calls will keep coming in.

For the child's parents, though, this is the day that will never be forgiven. The day of amputation, of powerlessness, of death. The day an earthquake tore a canyon in the ground and everything slipped from their grasp. Nothing will be the same again.

I cannot imagine how this feels. I don't want to try. How can they recover from this? Why would they even want to? This is who they are now: parents of loss. Recovery is the wrong word; the very thought an insult. Bereavement is not an illness to overcome. What is it, then? An emptiness? An explosion? A thousand futures imagined and none of them this.

Later they'll return to their silent home. They'll face the story of their lost child: the empty cot, the photographs, the bitter stockpile of surplus nappies and wipes. The appointments no longer needed; the floundering silent unbroken sleepless nights. In the chilling moment when there is nothing to be done but face their unconceived reality, what will they say and do? It is an empty question: I have no idea.

Once we're ready, we'll make ourselves available again, and we'll be sent to our next patient. It will be a woman who's got upset at her son's primary school and begun breathing fast and then felt dizzy, and either fallen or sat on the floor. She'll refuse to speak initially, rolling from side to side and clutching her head and her chest, and when she does speak, it will be to tell us she can't walk. And all the while we are gently reassuring her, and she is demonstrating her distress with her frowns and her whimpers, she will have no idea what our last job has been.

XXVII

I am a tourist. This is what I've become. A furtive rubber-necker, a short-haul confidant. Through years of abrupt, fleeting encounters. A connoisseur of private sentiment. A sightseer in a Teflon coat.

I drop into your misfortune, rummage around in your sacred chaos, take a mental snapshot, get my kicks out of handing out some assistance, then disappear off into the night, glad it's you and not me. My affinity with your experience is the blink of an eye, because I'm never here long enough to have to deal with any of your long-term struggles. Your crisis is my diversion, your mishap my anecdote, your tragedy my endeavour and my fulfilment. And then I'm gone.

The interactions of this job are intense, intimate and, once finished, consigned to the past. Not so much forgotten, but stripped of any investment or personal concern. The average patient contact is about an hour. Long enough to become acquainted, but no more than professionally involved; to empathise, within limits; to intervene, but never in the long term to have to commit. There are official boundaries to this

287

interaction, but there's also a more instinctive relational code to observe. I am kind and I am sympathetic and I am professional, and I am cold and I am heartless and I am protecting myself. None of this costs me anything beyond an occupational attachment, so long as there's no one involved here who will weigh on my mind.

It's a Saturday afternoon, ten days before Christmas. The biggest weekend in the season of excess. I'm at home trying to fix the toilet – the height of festivity – when I get the call.

Mum?

Sorry to bother you.

Is everything all right?

She never calls on a Saturday afternoon.

I'm not interrupting anything, am I?

It's fine. What's going on?

The hairs on my neck have stood to attention.

I'm at Liverpool Street.

Are you okay?

It's your dad.

You're at the station? What's happened?

I'm so sorry.

Is he okay?

We've had a bit of a problem. He's disappeared.

My dad was diagnosed with Alzheimer's a month before his sixtieth birthday. He'd been showing symptoms for a while, so who knows when the disease first started chipping away at his brain. From that moment on, this neural impostor became his second self, an uninvited companion that gradually undermined him until it had stolen his identity.

The initial changes took the form of subtle shifts rather than sudden plunges. We had noticed but not noticed and hoped for the best; sensed a change but looked for explanations elsewhere; detected an inward curve to his interactions, a door pulling itself closed on the outside world at an almost imperceptible speed.

In a cruel distortion of his easy-going nature, there was a new tendency towards frustration, a resentment of any kind of assistance, an exasperation with inanimate objects and anything novel or unfamiliar. Some of this felt like the stubbornness of ageing, but there was something more diminishing, more malignant to these personality shifts. He became preoccupied with written instructions, started creating *aides memoires* to help with daily tasks, began making tiny but significant miscalculations such as leaving the stove on or forgetting his way home in a town centre he knew well. The diagnosis simply confirmed what we already knew, and the long slow process of withdrawal began.

Because he was still young – still working, still active, still healthy, still involved – he became just about the most energetic dementia sufferer around. His days were characterised by a newfound restlessness, a muscular outworking of the pent-up infuriations of being trapped inside a body that could not process its experiences in the way it used to and still sensed it should be able to; a body that felt somehow barred from interactions it vaguely recognised but was unable to name or enact as it once could, so that it was always lagging behind, always peering through a frosted screen at events taking place too quickly. All of which manifested itself in pacing, in fiddling, in rifling through papers and realigning piles, in checking and rechecking, in tearing up documents into confetti fragments, in vigorously discarding, in marching rapidly in arbitrary directions, in movements that were purposeful and assertive but also haphazard and petulant and born of frustration and the need for a release, to find something, to get somewhere, anywhere. Add this to his slimline physique and his lifelong love of the outdoors and you had a potent combination: a man determinedly on a mission, unstoppable and spirited – but in pursuit of a goal he was temporarily unable to recall.

It's early evening when I reach the station, and the concourses are teeming with revellers, winter tourists and exhausted shoppers. Announcements squawk over the tannoy. Concertinaed shopping bags crash into shins, heels clatter on escalators, arms are flung round shoulders and shouts of sozzled affection are thrown back and forth. I weave through the pedestrian traffic on a different kind of quest, light-footed, single-minded, my eyes scanning rapidly in all directions, peering up platforms, round pillars and inside boutiques in search of my dad's white beard and distinctive blue coat. I feel like a foreigner, a creature operating in a separate reality and at a different speed.

He went missing from Boots, in the handful of seconds it took my mum to pay for a bottle of water. She turned around and that was it – he had vanished. That was two hours ago now.

Clearly, a major transport hub in a capital city is not the ideal place to lose somebody who's physically fit but functionally vulnerable. Liverpool Street hosts four Underground lines and countless overland routes; its surrounding roads, accessible from a multitude of exits, stretch out in all directions across the city. And this, of course, is one of the busiest days of the year.

We reconvene at the police station opposite, where my mum has made a report, given a description, offered any information that might be of use. The officers are kind, calm, professionally concerned. They tell us they'll do everything they can, but the station is hectic and they're clearly stretched.

Does your father carry a mobile phone?

He does . . . The problem is, he always turns it off. It's like a compulsion.

Any sort of GPS device?

Unfortunately not. He's quite resistant to stuff like that.

That's a shame. Something to think about. In the future maybe.

It's not a rebuke, but the implication hangs in the air, and we find ourselves answering the questions in an apologetic tone. It pushes the conversation in a different direction, where the procedural limits are set out and our expectations have been confined, managed. I'm used to being the relaxed professional in this exchange, not the one in need.

My sisters and brothers-in-law arrive with a car. We wonder where he's likely to have gone. It's possible he's followed some homing instinct and made for a familiar landmark, perhaps west towards the Barbican, Covent Garden or the West End, or maybe south for the river. It's a guessing game.

One of the quirks of the dementia is that it's hard to trace a train of thought. The brain finds connections which make sense only in retrospect. Has he been swept up in a crowd? Has he followed someone through the barriers and hopped on a Tube to a far-flung corner of the city? Has he simply tried to find somewhere quiet for a rest? The possibilities are almost limitless.

Four of us jump in the car and explore the more prominent nearby locations: hopping out, scouring the meandering streets, jumping back in, moving on. We sidestep carousers and theatre-goers, duck down alleys, peer through windows, show photos to bouncers outside bars. The police are check-ing the station CCTV, but this could take hours. Hours during which anything could be happening to him. In the meantime we will run our eyes across as many faces as we can, in search of that one cherished arrangement of flesh and bone.

Any degenerative disease slides imperceptibly from one phase to the next. In my dad's most active phase, we would walk with him to satisfy this energetic compulsion he had, to power onwards towards the horizon, as if he was trying to escape from something – perhaps the illness that was slowly withering his mind. We would take him to tree-filled parks or the landscaped gardens of stately homes, clinging to his past interest in horticulture. My mum would trudge with him across the fields near their house, or along the prom at the nearby coast, where he would walk and walk in silence, no longer initiating conversations, replying solemnly in ready-made epithets plucked instinctively from the distant past, delivered with a once-joyful face now trapped in a frown. This was a man who had been effusive and considerate, unassumingly sociable, dispensing reassurance in a gentle bass voice. Now he answered by rote, at great effort, I suspect, filling in the gaps to maintain the appearance of normality for as long as he could.

Another curious habit developed. For a short time he refused to walk by anyone's side. I once took him to the Botanical Gardens in Cambridge and he spent the whole day two or three paces behind me. When I stopped to let him catch up, he stopped too. If I slowed gradually until he was next to me, so we could at least imitate the gestures of famil-iarity, he too would slow and fall back behind. It sounds mildly pitiful to admit it, but over the course of the day this back-and-forth developed into a kind of contest between us: I was conscious of my responsibilities and keen to keep an eye on him, but he seemed almost childishly determined to retain some sort of independence by setting his own pace. It created a stilted, almost farcical stop-start dynamic to our day together, and short of turning round and walking back-wards, I struggled to keep him safe while allowing him his space. In the end I found a compromise by glancing over my shoulder every few paces and calling out cheerfully,

You okay, Dad?

What we had effectively created was a reversal in which I was the concerned, slightly impatient parent and my cheery, unflappable father had become a querulous child trying to prove a point. It was just another of the minor relational insults doled out by this slow-motion wrecking ball of a disease.

I make my way back to the station and set out again on foot. The others have gone home to make posters, to check on my mum, to chase up the police. They are doing the rational, pragmatic things: maximising resources. But I have decided to keep walking, maybe all night, to eliminate the streets one by one.

By now it's late evening and the night is mercifully dry. Cold, but not bitter. The crowds at the station are thinning out, some of the nearby pubs and bars are closing; others are just getting started. In the sociable groups that fill the pavements now, you'd think a white-haired former lawyer would stand out like a sore thumb. But of course, if he gives the appearance of having somewhere to go, if he's marching with his usual resolve, then he won't look so out of place. His body carries none of the signs of illness; he could easily pass unnoticed as a slightly quirky individual making his erratic way home.

I head east, through and around Spitalfields, towards Brick Lane, winding up and down the gridded streetmap to cover as much tarmac as I can, heel after toe, head turning left and right, eyes wide; then south towards Aldgate, Whitechapel, and east towards the Royal London hospital. As soon as I find one place that lacks him, I move on to the next.

I walk the main thoroughfares, tracing a perimeter, then turn back on myself into the side streets and fill in the gaps. I divert into shops, parks, Tube stations, bus stops and service yards. I wander up side alleys and round behind bins and inside stairwells and through underground car parks. It's amazing the number of places you can get into when you've got a good enough reason.

The places I go would be out-of-bounds on any other day, but today I'm wearing a cloak of invincibility, knowing he might be here, oblivious to any danger, vulnerable and alone. This boldness, a stranger to my normal self, makes me feel as if I'm taming the city, taking possession, renouncing its darkness.

I wander north to Bethnal Green and west to the nightlife of Shoreditch and Hoxton. People queue for entry to clubs, giggle and scream, stumble and are caught by their friends. They step in and out of the roads, cheering at passing mini-cabs, protected from danger by their youth and their beauty and their confidence. What would my dad make of all these people if he found himself here? Everyone I walk past is exuberant, invincible, possessed of endless tomorrows. I am in among them – and a thousand miles away.

I turn down a road past a hotel foyer (empty) and come across John Wesley's house and chapel beside the Museum of Methodism, anachronisms among this nightlife that would have fascinated my dad the preacher. But of course he's not here – such a coincidence would be too grand. The reality hits me afresh – he could be anywhere by now. What am I thinking?

I trace the geometry of the surrounding streets and work my way back down to Liverpool Street and the back entrances to the station. A vast zone of air outlets, industrial pipework and concrete seems to have potential as a refuge for the exhausted or the lost, and I slalom through the decorative shrubs, peering into the shadowy corners, but, again, there's no sign. I check the back exits to the station – perhaps he made his escape earlier through one of these doors? If only I could work out which.

I go west to the Barbican and its labyrinth of streets on stilts, then down to the illuminated dome of St Paul's – will its familiarity have drawn him to its steps for succour? Rest for the weary, comfort for the heavy-burdened? There's no sign. Then south, over the river and along the South Bank, into each of the brutalist monoliths facing the Thames – exactly the kinds of place he might find shelter, among reminders of a cultured past, a love of classical music, the theatre, the arts. But neither is he here.

The hours are ticking by. My initial vigour is waning. My feet ache. Am I beginning to lose hope? Perhaps my faith is misplaced. I feel sure that what I'm doing is worthwhile, but in a city woven with streets that stretch in all directions, crammed with endless houses and commercial buildings, throbbing and festive and anonymous and alive, do I seriously expect to be able to locate one human being among the several million others who are happily going about their business?

I know the chances are small. But one of the truisms of my job is that while most of the population keeps its head down and never requires us, there are certain people who will always appear – the regulars, of course, but also the helpless who are somehow caught in one of the colloquial safety nets of human vigilance, or simply show up when all hope seems lost. My conclusion has to be that the impossible numbers lie, and we are not as invisible as we sometimes seem. There may be thousands of streets, but with every one of them I walk down I shorten the odds.

At dawn, having walked straight through the night, I head home, the soberest passenger on the morning train, and sleep until lunch. When I wake there is news.

In among hours of CCTV playback, the police have found footage of a man in a bright blue coat boarding a Metropolitan line train bound for Uxbridge. There's only one thing to do. My wife and I leave the kids with a friend and drive there. I don't know what we think we'll find.

By now hope is waning. He's been missing for over twenty hours. Apart from the fact we don't know where he is, we have no idea what he's been doing – is doing now. Has he sat down to rest? Fallen? Collapsed? Is he injured? Has he slept, and if so where? Has he had anything to eat or drink? He has no money. Would he think to buy a drink even if he did? Would some primal need overtake him? Has he been approached by anyone? Attacked or exploited? These are not things we want to think.

Racked with guilt, my mum is convinced the next thing we'll hear is that a body has been found. We tell her it's too early to think like that, but with every hour that passes this possibility shuffles into view.

We must stay positive, we tell each other and ourselves. He's not entirely vulnerable. Could the urge to march off at speed be the same instinct that now keeps him safe?

My sisters and brothers-in-law have begun putting posters around the city. We are now those people: the family taping up swollen photocopies of snapshots in desperation. I find the idea horrible, exposing, shameful. The police tell us their investigations are ongoing. They're working through other footage, sending out details, and arranging a public appeal.

This is what it feels like on the other side, I realise, where the calm reassurances dispensed by the emergency services ring hollow because your mind is busy churning all the possible disasters. To the professional, it's a question of discharging one's duty, no more and no less, so that you can go home in the knowledge you have done all you can. But to the family, it might be a matter of life and death.

I've been in their position myself, answering all the anxious queries with the standard reassuring slogans, and now I'm hearing them rather than saying them, they sound uncomfortably close to nonchalance. It's a moment of enlightenment for me amid the drama – how easily the practised platitudes are dispensed; how empty they can sound.

When we get to Uxbridge, we look around the station for any trace. We know he got on a train bound this way, but did he make it this far? My wife appeals to the station supervisor for help – and something she says works: we're whisked into a side office and sat in front of a line of screens. We know when he got on, so try to work out when that train would have arrived here. The supervisor shows us footage of the exit gates and the platform from yesterday. The train spills out its passengers, the platform fills, then slowly empties. There's no sign of him. He didn't get this far.

But then I get a shock.

I look to my left, and not half a metre from where I've been sitting for the last twenty minutes is a crumpled pile of bright blue cloth. There's a tiny implosion in my chest. It's the right colour. I can see a zip. It's a coat.

Sorry. Do you know what this is here?

That's where they leave the lost property. Recognise something?

Do you mind if I have a look?

Be my guest. Probably picked up off the train.

I lift it up. I unfold it. I put my hand in the pockets – and find my dad's gloves.

It's a lightning bolt. I feel suddenly energised, impatient, unsure quite what to do with myself. There's a pang of urgency, a little illusion of proximity because I'm holding the item he was wearing when he disappeared. I call my family and tell them: we've found his jacket; I have it in my hand.

We learn that the jacket was collected from a seat during the litter pickers' sweep, which means he disembarked somewhere between Liverpool Street and here. There are nineteen stops, and nineteen miles, between the two stations, and that was a short lifetime ago. As astonishing as the moment is, it doesn't get us much closer to our goal.

It feels like Uxbridge has nothing left to offer us, so we head to the nearby hospitals to ask if any unnamed patients have been brought in yesterday or today. No joy.

Sat outside the last of them, I call work to tell them I won't be in for my shift in the morning. I explain what's happened, and ask if they can arrange for the ambulance service in

London to issue a missing-persons message to their crews. My manager takes the description, and we start the drive home. It's getting dark by now, and the prospect of my dad being missing for a second night is suddenly very real. This feels like a killer blow.

I speak to the police again to find out if anything's changed. For all their reassurances and professionalism, I feel like an inconvenience for asking. I'm the unrealistic family member trying to will something to change, unable to face reality. There's no news.

We're now due to make an appeal on the radio tomorrow, and by a process of elimination it looks like it's me who'll do the talking. When I get home I start thinking about what to say. I make a few notes to make sure there's nothing I'll miss: his appearance, his vulnerability, the number to call.

As I sit at the kitchen table, the tiredness of the previous night's walking catches up with me and I'm suddenly shorn of all hope. I wonder where he is and what's happening to him right now. Is he somewhere cowering in fear? Confused, hungry, alone? Is anyone with him? Why has no one reported a sighting?

I see my long night of trudging the streets for what it was: not a heroic act of defiance or dedication, but a cowardly refusal to accept the truth. Not just that my dad has vanished and is beyond my reach, utterly vulnerable and lost. And not just that I'm powerless to save him; that with the greatest determination in the world, all my efforts have fallen short. But also that these truths apply just as brutally to the illness that has taken over his brain.

I thought if I kept him active I could stave off the confusion. I thought if I kept his mind occupied it would halt the decline. By refusing to discuss the dementia, I thought I could deny its power over our lives. I thought I could make the journey about something else.

And finally, I thought against the odds I could find him, and rescue him. But I was wrong.

For the first time in many hours, I don't know what to do. And then my phone rings.

Jake?

Yes . . .

It's work. Why are they calling? Am I in trouble?

We've had a call from the control room in London. There's a crew in west London. Jake, they've found your dad.

They call Alzheimer's a disease of the memory, but its real target is the character. It attacks and transforms and diminishes the personality, and takes over the space it's created, until there's little room left for the sufferer to call their own.

I used to think of it as a thief. A cuckoo that had robbed my dad of his dignity. Crushed his vitality. Extinguished the pilot light of generosity in his heart. I used to think the dementia had stolen his love of life.

But the truth is something different. The truth is, it couldn't — because he'd already given it all away. He had shared his kindness with those around him. He had bestowed his wisdom and his humour on his family and friends. He had bequeathed his passions to his children and grandchildren — his love of travel and thrillers and music and words — and walking; his faithfulness and his faith. He had been doing this all his life. Long before the dementia first got its claws into him, and long after it had done its worst, he had hidden his humility and his joy in our hearts.

A woman in Shepherd's Bush looks out of her window and spots a man loitering by her front wall. She waits to see if he moves on, but he doesn't seem to know which way to go. She goes outside and asks him if he's okay. He's confused, lost, but able to tell her his name and that he used to work in a church. With some difficulty, she persuades him to come inside, then gives him a drink and calls 999.

By special request, the ambulance crew takes him to my sister's house in south London. My mum has been sleeping, finally, after the longest night and day of her life. When the ambulance arrives, they are reunited. My dad is tired, but clean, uninjured, safe. He seems bemused by all the attention.

He has been gone for twenty-eight hours, and crossed from one side of London to the other, and we will never know where he's been or what has happened to him along the way.

XXVIII

A new illness transforms the working lives of ambulance crew

Can You Hear Me? was first published in early 2020, just as the coronavirus crisis was emerging. Within weeks, the newly identified disease Covid-19 had transformed the working lives of ambulance crews. In this additional chapter for the new edition, I offer a few insights into the initial response.

It starts with a cough. *M'hem-b'hem!* Another, and another, from behind the door. *H'khhum, h'khhum, h'khhum!* A rhythmic bark of annoyance, a muffled expulsion of air. Sometimes a gasp. This is the last of four night shifts, and I've been hearing this sound all week: the dry relentless scraping of the voice-box, the clawing at an irritant that can't be moved. It's 4.15 a.m., and my eyes are dry and heavy, and our final patient is making the familiar sound.

I think he's up against the door.
Has he spoken to you?
I can hear him groaning.
What time did he fall?
About nine o'clock.

303

He's been there for seven hours.

I turn the handle and push at the door, and his wife's right; the solid wood comes up against his head.

What's the gentleman's name?

Graham.

I speak into the door.

Graham? I need to open the door. Can you move your head even slightly for me?

I push slowly but firmly. There's no other way to do this. I hear a groan, then another cough. The door yawns creakily to about eight inches: the width of my head. I turn my shoulders and slide my head through the gap and twist and take in the scene. A small bedroom with a mechanical bed. A medical over-table. A Zimmer. The scattered detritus of illness – crumpled tissues and blankets and greasy half-glasses of water. The stale aroma of quarantine. Ammonia, sweat. And a heavy, heaving figure in hospital pyjamas, prone and breathless, wedged against the door.

I slide my body through the gap. I'm outfitted in a mask, a gown, goggles and gloves: a faceless figure from a sci-fi film. I shout my words; they're muffled by my mask:

It's the ambulance! I need to move you away from the door!

I check Graham's head and neck, then take his legs, one under each arm, as if we're about to enter the world's most ill-advised wheelbarrow race, and heave him backwards across the sticky carpet. The pyjama top rides up to his armpits as I drag him away from the door. He coughs and coughs, a humourless laugh: *M-huh-huh-hurgh!* His mask dangles around his neck, not covering any part of his face.

My crewmate follows me into the room. It's late March and this is our new normal. A month ago, Covid-19 was a hazy villain looming on the horizon; a nasty rumour we hoped had been overhyped. Now its physical reality is everywhere we look, an acquaintance that follows us wherever we go.

Our patient is a man in his late seventies who's fallen in his bedroom and has clearly been coughing into the carpet through the dark of the night. We were told en route that he's confirmed positive and recently been discharged from hospital. He is flushed and floppy and short of breath. He's the battered finale of a gruelling week.

In spring 2020 a new type of patient began presenting to the ambulance service. We were used to dealing with breathing problems, but there was something different about the Covid-19 patients. They'd had the cough and the fever and the muscle aches, and after a week or so they'd start to feel better. Then the breathlessness hit them and they'd plummet. We'd turn up about ten days in, called for chest tightness, and they'd be sitting on their sofas talking to us, the TV on mute, breathing a little faster than normal, explaining calmly how a trip to the toilet was like climbing a mountain. And we'd put the sats probe on their fingers and discover they were acutely, even critically oxygen-deprived. You'd never know to look at them how unwell they were, how much damage had already occurred in their lungs. How could patients who were so short of oxygen appear so relaxed? Why weren't their chests heaving in great bucketfuls of air? Their hearts racing? Why weren't their bodies desperately trying to compensate?

This was a deceptive kind of hypoxia: an attack so subtle the victim didn't know it was happening. The parallels were clear. This new disease had stolen in under the guise of something altogether less sinister.

For about a month our job became a simpler, crueller, more streamlined version of itself. The low-acuity jobs disappeared, and almost everyone was ill with the same thing: it was just a case of determining where each patient sat on the Covid spectrum. Some were holding up well and could be left at home with self-care advice; others needed to be scooped up and whisked off to hospital for high-level interventions within minutes of arriving. Fleetingly, we were doing the job we'd always imagined: encountering critically ill patients, intervening decisively and providing rapid transport to definitive care. You'd never say things were better this way, but there was an intrinsic momentum in being needed. In the energised apparatus of a major incident unfolding in real time, we found ourselves gliding around with absolute clarity of purpose.

Sometimes the calls came in as something else entirely: diabetic problems or a stroke because of the confusion; even psychiatric issues when the lack of oxygen made patients antagonistic. Again and again we received messages saying patients were 'Covid-unlikely', only to turn up and find they had the full range of symptoms and were extremely unwell. We were learning as we went, less via official channels and more from what we'd seen out on the road or heard about from colleagues. The illness was novel, and the guidebook we had was only generically useful. The specifics emerged unannounced: the initial recovery followed by a second, more perilous wave of sickness; the silent hypoxia; the loss of taste and smell; the worrying prevalence of secondary blood clots. News of these characteristics was passed around mess rooms and taken into account before official advice had caught on.

We frequently went into rooms where unmasked patients had been coughing freely for days: hothouses of disease, where every surface was dusted with contagion, and the air itself felt like a portentous fog. Many of our colleagues were off sick with fevers and coughs – was this how they'd succumbed? We gave patients face coverings, and packaged them up before a trip to hospital, but our initial assessments and treatments took place in environments that were often highly infectious. Proffering a mask, I asked one patient if he'd had a cough recently. By way of answer, in a kind of instinctive response, he coughed full in my face. Others pulled their masks down to splutter throatily, then pulled them back up afterwards, and one woman refused to put a mask on at all. I explained that we couldn't treat her until she did, and a standoff ensued: was she being difficult, or was something physiological making her behave this way? Under the Covid cloud, the standard interactions carried an extra tension.

Some days were brutal: a succession of patients deteriorating in front of us; the suspicion that, for many, their call or our response had come too late; an echoed lament, fresh and unique with each encounter, of fear and loss. The nature of our job meant we never faced a ward full of critically ill patients and the promise of more on the way. For ambulance crews, the scale of devastation was witnessed in repetition, the numbers slowly adding up. There were shifts when we pulled out an oxygen mask for almost every patient, and delivered each of them to a resus department filled with nodding, vacant figures with faraway eyes and futuristic masks strapped to their faces, slumped on trolleys constantly being shuffled around to make room for new arrivals, before wiping down every inch of the ambulance and making ourselves available to do the same thing all over again, knowing full well what the next call would be. It was hard to escape the sense, during those early weeks, that we were fighting a losing battle.

I remember waiting in a corridor to hand over a patient on oxygen, surrounded by other crews with patients in the same predicament: a line of previously healthy people with newly inadequate lungs. A few weeks earlier, these cases would have been some of the first on the list, but now there was a fresh and ruthless hierarchy in play, so they waited. Patients already assessed and admitted dragged around personal bottles of oxygen on little trolleys, stopping to rest every few steps. We were in an oxygen-dependence farm, and it was completely routine. When people suggested the crisis had been overstated, or neighbours had friends round for lockdown barbecues, or people said it was time for things to 'get back to normal', this was the scene I wanted them to see.

One of the tougher new realities was that relatives were banned from hospital. Out in the community, as the link between home and hospital, it fell to ambulance crews to tell patients they had to make this frightening journey alone. Any mention of coronavirus carried distressing associations, naturally, and patients wanted a familiar face to comfort and reassure them. Family members in turn were desperate to look out for their loved ones and advocate on their behalf amid the maelstrom of medicalised endeavour, and we felt guilty for dragging them apart.

One day we transferred an elderly woman from a local clinic to A&E. She spoke almost no English and was weak and short of breath. Just before we left, her son arrived and stepped onto the ambulance. We told him he wouldn't be allowed to come, but that the hospital would call to update him. There was no way to know what was going to happen to her, but he clearly understood the possibilities, and I felt how inadequate the moment was, how banal and chaotic, in this strange cramped setting, as he reached round our tangle of wires to hug her and lingered for a second before climbing down the steps and shutting the door as we put on our lights and disappeared.

I think of Graham a week later when I'm watching the news. There's a report from the intensive care unit at University College Hospital London. It shows the clinicians turning an intubated, comatose patient onto their front to aid their breathing. The process is delicate and time-consuming and involves eight members of staff.

We have to do something similar with Graham here: he's been lying on his front for seven hours. We need to roll him onto his back, then get him off the floor and work out if he needs to return to hospital. My suspicion is he does. There are some differences: Graham is weak but conscious and he's not hooked up to a host of monitors and life-sustaining machinery. But he's also at floor level, in a cramped room full of obstacles and debris, and lacking any cooperative tone: a dead weight. He's sweaty and dishevelled and breathing rapidly, and soaked in urine and actively coughing. And big. And there are only two of us here.

We've asked for an extra pair of hands. Our dispatcher says they'll send a colleague on a car, but five minutes later we're told that resource has been sent on a cardiac arrest and there's no one else. We'll be doing this on our own.

This is the theme of our recent shifts. The service I work for has never been so busy. The public reticence about going to A&E is not extending to those phoning 999. Each day we're getting nearly twice the usual number of calls, and there's also a record number of staff off sick. Some patients, Graham included, are waiting a very long time for a response. No one we've been to has complained: they understand the pressure we're under; but that's not the point.

We check for injuries, slide Graham's arm under his torso and rotate him at the shoulders and hips. He rolls slowly and we ease him onto his back. *Cough, cough, cough, cough.* We sit him up, but he has no strength so it's more like pivoting a piece of unwieldy furniture. His body slumps to the side, so we slide him across the floor and spin him and rest his back against the bed. It's getting warm in here. We place a pillow behind his head and shoulders. His right arm is flaccid. Has he had a stroke? Is that why he fell? Or is it floppy because he's been lying on it all night? His flesh is a Rorschach of blotches where he's been pressed against the floor, the wall, the door.

How are you feeling, Graham? Do you have any pain?

He mumbles something about his arm. The toilet. A drink. Then a stumbling rallentando of throat-clearance. We fetch him some water. His breathing is rapid and shallow. We're trying to keep people at home if we can, but Graham clearly needs to go in.

We chat to him casually, as if we're here to play cards, as if we're not wrestling him around his bedroom, as if we normally dress like this, but he looks straight through us: there's something distant in his bearing, as if part of him has been expended during the night, and he can't see our faces behind these masks to read any reassurance, or even the exhaustion we're struggling to hide. He is mainly, now, a physical project.

We bend his knees and wedge his feet into his slippers, flat on the floor. We crouch either side and hook our arms and clutch at his sodden waistband, and stand him to an approximation of vertical. He has no power in his legs and needs to sit down. I give him a hug, his chin on my shoulder, his arms wrapped around me, while my crewmate grabs the carry chair, and we spin and deposit him and wrap around the blanket and strap. We wheel him to the stair-lift and repeat the process in reverse. The sweat is running down my back. And Graham's still coughing.

By the time we're at hospital we've lifted him five times like this, bracing and heaving upwards and swivelling and stretching and easing back down. The manoeuvres are awkward and restricted: the moving and handling department would be having a hernia if they could see us now. Who knows if our PPE was designed with this in mind? But this is the reality of pre-hospital care: a level of improvised proximity you can't exactly plan for, because there's always another detail to throw into the mix.

Personal protective equipment became an emotive public issue around this time. The contribution of frontline health workers was being recognised and celebrated in a way I'd never witnessed before, and when reports emerged of problems with the availability and suitability of protective gear, this only emphasised the apparent bravery and sacrifice of these newly- appointed champions. Social media campaigns raised funds and collected outraged signatures. Unions expressed formal concerns. In my ambulance service, we knew of (but didn't tell our families about) colleagues in intensive care with Covid-19.

Then the first healthcare worker deaths were reported. It was a moment that would soon be repeated to the point of guilty familiarity, but that initial shock registered like a dull heat in the centre of the chest. Of course, the deaths of health workers and the problems with PPE were not a single issue, but in those anxious early weeks, when staff were emotionally fragile and physically drained, such news only heightened people's frustrations and fears. Things were getting very real.

Every health worker had their own stories about PPE. I never experienced an acute shortage, so my concerns related more to suitability. This was a more nuanced issue than supply, because of the complex variety of interactions and responses occurring across the health service at the time.

While acknowledging the importance of local adaptation, the guidance from Public Health England focused on the clinical aspects of the patient encounter: what to wear for which clinical intervention. But ambulance work doesn't happen in a hospital cubicle; it's as much contextual as clinical, and some of what I wore felt ill-suited to the peculiar settings of my role. In our encounter with Graham, and a hundred others like it, the level of risk was determined neither by the severity of symptoms nor the interventions performed, but by the physical nature of the interaction and the chaotic environment in which it took place.

The aprons we wore, as part of our standard PPE for suspected or confirmed Covid-19 patients, epitomised this mismatch. During the initial outbreak, I wore a variety of plastic aprons, depending on availability. Some felt robust; others were as flimsy as the second-rate bin liners you might buy from the supermarket if you weren't concentrating, and would split if they caught on the radio on your belt. But the bigger problem was that they were a piece of attire clearly designed for indoor use. Remember the scene in *American Beauty* with the plastic bag dancing around in the alleyway? This was our problem: often as we walked out into the street, perhaps wheeling a breathless patient in the carry chair, the wind would catch the loose 'skirt' flap of material and whip it upwards: any infectious droplets shielded from your trousers would then be deposited on your chest or even face.

I began to wonder why I was wearing the aprons at all: rather than protecting me, their billowing excitability surely increased the risk of transmission. It gradually dawned on me that I was wearing the aprons because I felt I had to – my own submissive tribute to the philosophy that it's sometimes less important to do the right thing than to be *seen* to do the right thing. If I'd ever known for sure my apron had been contaminated, I would have removed it straightaway.

But behind the practical discussions about PPE lay a more profound question. What level of risk were we expecting our healthcare workers to accept? Should frontline staff be willing to accept *any* increased risk of infection compared with the general public? If so, how much – and why? When government statements assured us they were happy with the level of PPE, what exactly did this mean? Had some 'reasonable' level of extra risk been factored into this analysis? Was a figure ever discussed?

In a work context, surely the minimum requirement of PPE would be to reduce any extra risk associated with the work to a marginal figure? In other words, clinicians and carers encountering multiple Covid patients each day should be no more likely to contract the virus than a non-patient-facing manager sat at a desk. Yet, if this was the case, why were vulnerable colleagues being removed from patient-facing duties? This was surely a tacit admission that the level of protection was insufficient.

I couldn't locate any official discussion of this. For all the concern and public debate, I never heard a politician being asked what extra level of risk it was deemed appropriate for the nation's healthcare workers to place themselves under in the current crisis.

★

Easter weekend we work a run of early shifts. Coming in over the holiday feels less of a sacrifice because there's so little going on elsewhere. There's concern about patients avoiding A&E, but we're called to plenty of non-Covid emergencies: a stroke, a heart attack, a teenager with an arm fracture and a woman who's fallen in the garden and given herself some nasty facial injuries. There are signs the pre-hospital world's beginning to move out of the Covid storm.

Our last job on Sunday is to a care home for a patient with dementia and multiple ongoing conditions, but nothing that demands hospital right now. He's settled and comfortable, and we think he's better off staying here. We speak to his family over the phone, and they're happy to follow our advice, so we go out to the ambulance to complete our paper-work, to make a referral to an out-of-hours GP, to wipe all our equipment down. By the time all this is done we're well past the end of our twelve-hour shift.

When we go back into the care home with the paperwork and the referral details, the manager tells us they're about to call for another ambulance. They've got a second patient – is there any chance we could see them? Or do we already have another job?

To be honest, we've just finished our shift.

Oh, of course.

We can certainly come and see the patient, but you should still phone it through so they can get someone else running.

This call came at the end of a week when admiration for NHS staff was at its pinnacle. Radio shout-outs, hand-painted rainbows, newspapers testimonies, even a prime minister's tribute: you'd have been forgiven at this point for thinking the crisis was more about health workers than the disease itself. No doubt the fight against coronavirus was a more encouraging narrative than the simple facts of the devastation it was wreaking.

Out on the road, we'd experienced our own examples of appreciation: clapping as we drove past on blue lights; food donations delivered to our station; patients expressing their gratitude even when they'd waited ages for us to arrive. It was all a bit disconcerting when you're more accustomed to friction and even abuse. We were once parked up assessing a patient in the ambulance when the Thursday evening applause began all around us. It felt both uplifting and embarrassing. I waited until everyone had gone back into their houses and the coast was clear before sneaking round to the cab and driving off without any fanfare.

Now we grab some of our kit and follow the carers up to the second patient's room. She's a squat woman in an armchair, breathing rapidly, a half-smile on her face, as if she's remembering a funny story from long ago. My crewmate does a FAST test: the patient's speech is slow and she's unable to follow commands. But we've seen these symptoms a lot recently: we check the patient's oxygen levels and they're worryingly low. She's also got a high fever. Yes, it's possible she's had a stroke, but it's more likely that she's got Covid-19 and her confusion is due to an acute lack of oxygen reaching her brain. Her body's struggling to do its job on its own.

What felt odd about all the applause and the acclaim was that we weren't doing anything new. Perhaps from the outside, things looked very different; perhaps the reality of dealing with numerous Covid patients each day was hard to imagine, so people defaulted to assumptions of courage and endurance. But I didn't feel that I was being any braver or more caring than normal. The work had changed in that we were wearing PPE, and the focus of the wider health service had altered, and of course there was an extra risk involved. But the fundamental principles, of care and commitment, had not sprung up in response to coronavirus: they'd been there all along. The choices staff were making, across the NHS – to sit with a patient beyond the end of shift, to miss out on family time because a job wasn't finished, to do an Easter egg hunt in the dark when you got home because you were in the wrong (right) place at the wrong (right) time – were not rare feats of heroism reserved for an exceptional period of national turmoil; they were the routine acts of a workforce whose daily business is care.

The manager tells us she's made the 999 call for another ambulance, but we can see this patient shouldn't have to wait: she needs to go now. My crewmate looks at me and we know what we need to do.

I'll get the bed.

She takes her radio off her hip to tell Control we'll take the job ourselves.

Epilogue

The one thing you're not allowed to say on an ambulance is that you're here because you want to make a difference. Such sentiment is off limits, *verboten*, not the done thing at all. When I was brand new, an old-timer asked me:

So what made you want to do this then?

Before I could answer, he followed the question with a warning:

And don't say it's because you want to help people.

In this business, that would be like a child admitting they enjoy school: it might be true, but that doesn't mean you have to advertise the fact.

Instead, a kind of robust modesty becomes the order of the day: a stubborn embargo on egotism and conceit. Don't get above your station, don't use medical jargon, don't go thinking of yourself as a hero. And don't, whatever you do, wear your stethoscope around your neck.

But this self-deprecation is its own brand of pride, and I think we're in danger of selling ourselves short. Because we're all here to improve patient outcomes – to lift, to comfort, to deliver, to mend. We may not always get to perform the version of the job we envisaged, but we are participating in the communal matrix, and this is somehow the stuff of life.

For all the frozen entitlement of the contemporary world, there's something that compels human beings, in that critical moment when they see someone in need, to intervene – to go the extra mile for the stranger at the gate. This frustrating, rewarding, exhausting job is nothing more than a formalised enactment of that impulse: to answer the call for help, to remove someone from harm, and to take them to a place where the restoration can begin.

And, if the tables were turned, this is surely what any of us would want done for us.

Author's Note

It should be clear that this book is not a rehashing of clinical guidelines or an exemplar of best practice. Those with a clinical eye or time in the job may object to the occasions when things are not done strictly by-the-book, but I have tried to resist the urge to correct my actions with hindsight or add a layer of retrospective sugar-coating. I've also attempted to present the relevant context: ambulance crews don't work in consulting rooms, laboratories or classrooms (unless they're called to them); they work in the real world and make choices in real time. For those who feel the described actions reflect badly on the profession, I apologise: any errors are mine alone.

It should also be noted that clinical guidelines change with time, and this book spans a period of approximately ten years, during which there have been changes that may make aspects of the treatment seem outdated. I've tried to keep these anachronisms to a minimum to avoid confusion, while remaining honest about what was said and done at the time.

Certain details and all names have been changed.

Acknowledgements

I'd like to express my gratitude to my many excellent colleagues in the ambulance service, a few of whom make brief appearances here; I hope they feel the book does some justice to their ongoing exploits. A nod also to my colleagues in the other emergency services and across the wider health care world: emergency care is a collaborative endeavour. I want to thank Lauren and everyone at Bell Lomax Moreton, for the support, expertise and calmness, and Ben and everyone at Quercus, for shaping my words into the best book they could become. A few people read early drafts and samples, and offered helpful pointers and words of approval, for which I'm very grateful. A special thanks to my mum and sisters for allowing me to tell my dad's story. And most of all, for their support in many more things than just the writing of this book, thanks to my amazing wife and three brilliant children.